WILD GOOSE QIGONG

WILD GOOSE QIGONG

Natural Movement for Healthy Living

by Hong-Chao Zhang

張 宏 超

YMAA Publication Center
Wolfeboro, NH USA

YMAA Publication Center
Main Office:
  PO Box 480
  Wolfeboro, NH, USA 02131
  800-669-8892 • info@ymaa.com • www.ymaa.com

20200326

ISBN:978159439780

Edited by James O'Leary
Cover design by Ilana Rosenberg

Publisher's Cataloging in Publication
(Prepared by Quality Books Inc.)

Zhang, Hong-Chao, 1954-
    Wild goose qigong : natural movement for
healthy living / by Hong-Chao Zhang. —1st ed.
    p. cm. —(Qigong—health & healing)
    Includes index.
    ISBN: 1-886969-78-7

    1. Ch'i kung. 2. Ch'i kung—China—History.
I. Title. I. Series.

RA781.8.Z53 2000   613.7'1
          QBI99-500557

Disclaimer:
The author(s) and publisher of this material are NOT RESPONSIBLE in any manner whatsoever
for any injury which may occur through reading or following the instructions in this manual.
The activities, physical or otherwise, described in this material may be too strenuous or dangerous
for some people, and the reader(s) should consult a physician before engaging in them.

Printed in USA

Table of Contents

Editor's Note

The color of the arrows (black or white) was chosen to maximize visibility, no other meaning is implied. Also, a dashed line indicates movement behind the body.

The author has chosen to follow the Chinese convention in this book for many of the photographs. The arrows of a particular photograph often anticipate the motion for the next movement.

Romanization of Chinese Words

This book uses the Pinyin romanization system of Chinese to English. Pinyin is standard in the People's Republic of China and in several world organizations, including the United Nations. Pinyin, which was introduced in China in the 1950s, replaces the Wade-Giles and Yale systems. In some cases, the more popular spelling of a word may be used for clarity.

Some common conversions:

Pinyin	Also Spelled As	Pronunciation
Qi	Chi	chē
Qigong	Chi Kung	chē kǔng
Qin Na	Chin Na	chǐn nǎ
Jin	Jing	jǐn
Gongfu	Kung Fu	göng foo
Taijiquan	Tai Chi Chuan	tǐ jē chüén

For more information, please refer to *The People's Republic of China: Administrative Atlas, The Reform of the Chinese Written Language,* or a contemporary manual of style.

About the Author

Hong-Chao Zhang was born on December 20, 1954, in Lankao County, Henan Province, People's Republic of China (P.R.C.). He began learning Chinese Martial Arts (Wushu or Gongfu) from Grandmaster Niansheng Wu in his hometown when he was young.

From 1971 to 1974, he learned Chinese medicine, acupuncture, and massage at Gaozhuang Hospital in Yangchen County while living with his older brother, Haichao Zhang, a surgical and Chinese Medicine doctor, and his sister-in-law, Xiulan Nie, a general doctor.

From 1974 to 1989, he learned most internal and external Wushu with Grandmasters Jing-Ming Wen and Yu-hua Liu. Both helped introduce the world to Chinese Martial Arts at the 11th Olympic Games in Berlin, 1936.

From September 1976 to February 1977 he learned Wushu with Mr. Jianhua Guo at Wuhan Institute of Physical Education, P.R.C. Also in 1977 he was a chief coach of the Xiao Gan Wushu Team, and a director of the Xiao Gan Wushu Championships in Hubei, P.R.C.

In 1978, he received a Bachelor of Arts Degree in Wushu from the Wuhan Institute of Physical Education in Wuhan, Hubei Province, People's Republic of China, and also served as one of the five founders of the Qigong Research Association there. Also in 1978, he received a graduation certificate from the Advanced Training Program of College Level Teachers of Wushu at the Beijing University of Physical Education. While there, he studied with Grandmaster Wen-Guang Zhang, also one of the martial artists who introduced the world to Chinese Martial Arts at the Olympic Games in Berlin.

In 1987, he received a graduation certificate in Sports Injury Treatment, Chinese Medicine, Massage, and Acupuncture at Attached Hospital, Wuhan Institute of Physical Education.

In 1988, Master Zhang received a Master of Arts Degree in Wushu at the Shanghai Institute of Physical Education, a diploma of Wushu Graduate Student from the Wuhan Institute of Physical Education, and a diploma from the Swiss Kung Fu Wushu Taijiquan Federation as a Wushu instructor. In 1989, he received a graduation certificate from the National Taijiquan Training Program of the National Wushu Association and Research Institute of Wushu at Beijing, where he learned the Chen, Yang, Wu, and Sun styles of Taiji from Masters Xiaowang Chen, Bingci Li, Zhenduo Yang, and Jianyun Sun.

Master Zhang has extensive teaching experience. He was an assistant professor of Wushu from 1978 to 1989 at the Wuhan Institute of Physical Education. In 1979, he taught self-defense, Qinna (joints lock), and Dianxue (acupuncture points) to the Hubei Province Police Organization.

From 1979 to 1980, he was an assistant professor of Wushu at two six-month seminars for Chinese university teachers of Wushu of the National Advanced University Wushu Training sponsored by the National Committee of Education, at the Wuhan Institute of Physical Education. Also instructing at these special seminars were Master Zhang's mentors, Grandmaster Jing-Ming Wen and Yu-hua Liu.

In 1989, Master Zhang traveled to the U.S. as a visiting professor and taught Wushu at Ball State University in Muncie, Indiana from 1989 to 1990.

From 1990 to the present, he has been teaching Wushu (Gongfu) at Truman College in Chicago, Illinois and also at his own studio in Chicago, Chinese Gongfu Institute. In 1991, he received a certificate from the United States Combat Wrestling Association. From 1992 to 1994, he was a part-time instructor of physical education and therapy at the Jeannine Schultz Memorial School in Park Ridge, Illinois. In 1993, he taught self-defense and Qinna to the Lake County Illinois Chiefs of Police Organization. In 1997, he started teaching Wushu at the University of Illinois at Chicago. In the same year, he was a technical advisor to the Organizing Committee of the Fifth Zhengzhou China International Shaolin Wushu Festival.

Since 1978, Master Zhang has published many articles in the People's Republic of China such as:

"Silian Quan," *Journal of Wuhan Institute of Physical Education*, No. 2, 1980.

"Wushu and Prolonged Life," *Journal of Wuhan Institute of Physical Education*, No. 4, 1981.

"Preliminary Analysis of Spring Force in Wushu," *Journal of Wuhan Institute of Physical Education*, No. 2, 1982.

"Injury and Prevention of Ischiadic Article," *Bianliang Wushu*, No. 4, 1983.

"Training of Technique of Boxing," *Translated Journal of Wuhan Institute of Physical Education*, No. 3, 1984.

"Training of Strategy and Tactics of Boxing," *Translated Journal of Wuhan Institute of Physical Education*, No. 1, 1985.

"Knowledge and Method of Wrap-up Binding of Boxing," *Translated Journal of Wuhan Institute of Physical Education*, No. 2, 1986.

"Preliminary Research on Forgetfulness of Movements in Teaching Wushu Patterns," *Journal of Wuhan Institute of Physical Education*, No. 3, 1986.

"Wushu is Entering the Olympic Games," *Shaolin Wushu*, No. 5, 1988.

In 1987, six undergraduate students of Master Zhang all received awards at the First National Conference on the Scientific Study of Wushu in Beijing, and Master Zhang's article, "Research and Review of all Wushu Magazines," received an award from the Wushu Research Institute of China and the Chinese Wushu Association. His book, *Handbook of Boxing*, was published in 1989 by Northeast Engineering University Publishing House, People's Republic of China.

Not only has Master Zhang published articles and books, but he has also received many honors. Before coming to the U.S., Master Zhang served as a judge and chief coordinator in over twenty national, local, regional, and university Wushu competitions. In 1978, he was one of the judges for a famous Hong Kong Gongfu movie star, Lianjie Li (known as Jet Li in the U.S.) at Chengde, Hebei Province. In 1985, he received an Excellent National Judge of Wushu Award and also was a National First Class Judge of Wushu. In 1986, he was a recipient of an Excellent National Teacher of Education Award.

In 1990, he was a winner, Black Belt Division, Kata, PKC National Tournament, Anderson, Indiana. In 1991, he was a winner in the Black Belt Competition "Battle of Chicago" Karate Championships. He also won in the Black Belt Competition, Winning Edge Karate Championships and the Black Belt, First Annual Chinese Martial Arts Open Competition held in Chicago. In 1993, he was a winner in Advanced Taiji, North American Chinese Martial Arts Federation Competition held in Baltimore, Maryland. In 1995, he won two gold medals in Advanced Chen Style Taiji and Advanced Other Style Taiji at the USA Chinese Martial Arts Open Championship in Mobile, Alabama. Also in 1995, he received a certificate for participating as a demonstrator in the 1995 World Wushu Championships in Baltimore, Maryland. He currently serves as an advisor to the USA Wushu Kung Fu Federation. He is the vice-president of the Chicago Chinese Council and the president of the Super International Trade Corporation. He is the president of the Henan Province Association of Chicago and a corporate advisor for new business development of Kraft Foods.

In 1997, Master Zhang was a competitor at the fifth Zhengzhou China International Shaolin Wushu Festival, where he was awarded exhibition prizes in short weapons and Chen Style Taiji, and a second place award in Taiji competition.

Foreword by Professor Yu-Hua Liu

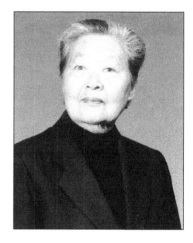

The author has asked me to write a few words about *Wild Goose Qigong*. Even though my expertise is in Wushu (Gongfu), I am glad to write a preface for this book. The reason is because this author, Hong-Chao Zhang, was one of my students in China. He always respected his teachers, and he is honest and tolerant and sincere with people. The heart of his undertaking is strong, and he has reached an exceptional level of skill in Wushu. For these reasons, my husband, Wen, Jing-Ming, and I chose him as our assistant professor to teach two special six-month seminars for all-China University teachers of Wushu in 1979 and 1980. The author was the best student of Professor Wen's later years, and he was the only graduate student teaching Wushu at the Wuhan Institute of Physical Education before 1988. He had been under the training of Professor Wen since 1974 and almost mastered all the theory and skill of Wushu. He always took Professor Wen (by bicycle!) to see the doctor when my husband was ill. Especially when Professor Wen stayed in the hospital during the last several months of his life, the author visited him every day and helped to care for him. After Professor Wen passed away, the author helped put the uniform on my husband's body and took him to the funeral parlor before cremation.

There was no other student like Hong-Chao Zhang in his dedication and kindness to my husband and me.

Second, the author studied diligently and trained hard. He learned Wushu from Professor Wen during many summer vacations. At the same time, he visited the foremost grandmasters of Wushu in China and trained under them also. Not only did he master the art of Wushu, but he also studied Qigong as well. He was one of the five founding members of the Qigong Research Association at the Wuhan Institute of Physical Education in 1980. He published many articles and a book on Wushu. Particularly, in 1985, after Meijuen Yang taught Qigong at our institute, he studied and trained hard. This book is the crystallization of his diligent study and hard training.

Wild Goose Qigong has beneficial effects on all the organs and systems of the human body. Practicing Qigong makes you feel younger and stronger. It prolongs life. In Chapter 4 of this book, the author not only gives you the training method of Wild Goose Qigong, but he also gives you the notes and effects of each movement, the acupressure points, and the channels to which they belong. It is a good book for people of all ages, from all walks of life, who want to train their discipline, improve their posture, flexibility, sensitivity, coordination, pliability, physical strength and fitness, concentration, attention, and meditations. The photos of this book and accompanying essays are excellent, making this book good for everyone who wants to learn about Qigong and achieve its benefits.

Yu-Hua Liu
Yu-Hua Liu is recognized as one of China's ten most famous Wushu Professors.

Preface

Although Qigong originated in China, it belongs to all the world. It is the wealth of the world.

Meijun Yang, my Wild Goose Qigong teacher, is over 104 years old, but she still practices Qigong every day and through its use treats patients who have difficult diseases. Wild Goose Qigong makes her much younger and stronger, and she has the secret solution to the riddle of prolonging life.

Wild Goose Qigong has good effects on all the organs and systems of the human body, such as the central nervous system, the cardiovascular system, the digestive system, and the respiratory system. It can also have positive effects on metabolism, cancer, and AIDS—and even on one's disposition. Practicing Wild Goose Qigong can also prevent and treat disease.

I started writing this book in Chinese at my leisure when I was teaching Chinese Martial Arts in the Department of Wushu at the Wuhan Institute of Physical Education in 1986. I continued to write this same book in English when I was teaching Chinese Martial Arts in the Physical Education Department at Ball State University in Muncie, Indiana in 1989. There, hundreds of students took my classes and earned two credits when they passed the test. My students learned self-defense; learned to train their discipline; improved their flexibility, sensitivity, coordination, and pliability; and improved their physical strength and fitness. Their most important benefits were improvements in concentration, attention, and meditation, from which they derived more energy to apply to their other studies.

Practicing Qigong is not limited by one's age or sex, where one practices, the weather, season, or time. It does not require any equipment. In general, you can, according to your schedule, practice at home, in the park, by the lake, in the forest, at the school, and so on. But no matter where you choose, the more peaceful the environment, the better.

In completing this book, I am greatly indebted to Mr. David Hoehne for proof-reading my first drafts, and to Ms. Suzy Byrne, who assisted me greatly with many preparatory photographs. My thanks also go to Ms. Laura Coats, who typed up the first manuscript. All gave great support in the fulfillment of this book. I would like to express my thankfulness for everyone's help.

Hong-Chao Zhang 張宏超
December, 1998

CHAPTER ONE

Introduction to Qigong and Wild Goose Qigong

1.1 INTRODUCTION TO QIGONG

Qigong is a way of life that combines the spirit, the physical body, and the breath, trained under the direction of consciousness. It functions as health maintenance, intellectual and life development, and physical strength training. The training involves gesturing, relaxation, mental concentration, a deeply concentrated, peaceful mind, breath control, movement of the limbs, and massotherapy.

The content of Qigong study is abundant and diverse. Based on the characteristics of the movements, it can be classified as Jing gong, which is static outside and moves inside; Dong gong, which has inner stillness throughout the movements; and Jing-dong gong, which combines both Jing gong and Dong gong. Based on an exercise's posture pattern (or form of training), it can be classified as Wogong (including lying down on the back or lying on one's side); Zuogong (including Duan zuo, which is sitting upright; Guizuo, which is sitting on your knees; Juzuo, which is sitting on one leg with your legs crossed and squatting down; and Dunzuo, which is squatting down with your feet parallel); Zhangong, Huobugong, and their combinations.[1] Based on an exercise's consciousness goals, it can be classified as Neishidantian (concentrating on your Dantian with your eyes closed), Cunshiwuzang (concentrating on your heart, liver, spleen, lungs, and kidneys), Cunnian (focusing your consciousness), and Yinqi (letting your mind lead your Qi). When classifying these exercises according to the breathing methods, you count the number of breaths (inhalation and exhalation). Based on the results of the training, the exercises can be classified as medical Qigong, health care Qigong, strength Qigong, etc.

The historical development of Qigong has produced the following five arts: health care Qigong, Ru Family Qigong, Dao Family Qigong, Shi Family Qigong, and Martial Arts (or Wushu) Qigong. There are different contents, forms, and characteristics of each family's Qigong.

Chinese Qigong has recently undergone vigorous growth as an academic topic. There are even new methods of practicing Qigong, including Guo Lin's "New Qigong Method," Ma Litang's "Knack of Six Words," Lian Shifeng's "Automatically Play the

Game of Five Animals," Wang Yufang's "Yi Quan Zhan Zhuang" (Consciousness by Standing), Zhao Jinxiang's "Chinese Hexiang Zhuang Qigong" (Crane Qigong), Yan Xin's Qigong, Zhang Zhitong's "Waidan Gong," Tian Ruisheng's "Modern Xiang Gong," Yang Meijun's "Wild Goose Qigong," and many, many more.

1.2 INTRODUCTION TO WILD GOOSE QIGONG

If Qigong is like a garden, then Wild Goose Qigong is like a beautiful flower. Wild Goose Qigong originated in Sichuan Province, with the famous instructor Dao An. Before Dao An there was only Fu An and the originator of Qigong, Hua Tuo (?–208 B.C.). Following Dao An was Wan Yi, the master monk of Wutai Mountain; he arranged and preserved Wild Goose Qigong, and it spread throughout China until the time of the Qing Dynasty. It is called Kunlun School Qigong. Wild Goose Qigong, which emphasizes action, adopts the method of natural breathing and is easy to learn and practice. With consistent practice over a long time, it can cure and prevent sickness, improve health and lengthen life. Because of this, it is also considered to be a form of Medical Qigong.

Wild Goose Qigong is a moving Qigong, imitating the form and movements of the wild goose found in nature. The movements of Wild Goose Qigong are beautiful, combining solid and soft qualities. They guide the movement of Qi in the body, circulating it in the twelve channels, and balancing Yin and Yang. Wild Goose Qigong has the characteristics of both static and dynamic disciplines, with the balance on the side of stillness. It emphasizes practicing and adjusting naturally. People who practice it must concentrate, quiet the mind, close the mouth naturally, touch the tongue to the palate, and relax the body, while attempting to move like a wild goose living in nature. Wild Goose Qigong doesn't emphasize breathing and consciousness—as long as one relaxes the whole body. Persistent practice can achieve the integration of consciousness, breath, and body.

Wild Goose Qigong contains the pre-64 form, the pro-64 form, Kunlun Chan Shou Bagua, Bazi Bayao Gong, and dynamic Qigong, etc. The pre-64 form is the basic; all others start from it. It is divided into 64 phases. This book introduces the pre-64 form first because of Wild Goose Qigong's medical and health value.

CHAPTER TWO

The History of Qigong

2.1 QIGONG IN REMOTE ANTIQUITY (26TH CENTURY B.C.–17TH CENTURY B.C.)

Chinese Qigong has a long history, which started at Taotang shi, Rao's tribal society (26th–22nd Century B.C.). At that time, people suffered from stagnation of Qi and blood, and tired muscles and bones, due to rain, floods, and cold, humid weather. They did exercises to improve their blood circulation.

Ancient people used to celebrate their memorial, hunting, and harvest ceremonies by imitating animals' jumping and flying in dance. The movements of the dances were guided by the movements of animals, such as climbing, looking, and flying. Qigong was a product of the struggle ancient people had with difficult environmental conditions and disease. This was a kind of original Qigong.[2] Just as Fu Yi in the East Han Dynasty explained the function of dance movements in Dance Verses:

> Dancing is an eternal skill to entertain one's spirit and slow down the process of getting old.

2.2 QIGONG DURING THE SHANGZHOU DYNASTY (17TH CENTURY B.C.–256 B.C.)

There were some wars during the Shangzhou Dynasty. People had to contend not only with difficult natural environments, but also with injuries and lack of adequate food. In order to cope with these hardships, people developed techniques based on their own experience—such as resting with closed eyes, self-massage, lightly patting the body, deep breathing, stretching, moving the body, and pressing the chest and abdomen—to fight disease without doctors and medicine. Learning through experience, they passed on these practices from generation to generation.

Yu Pie Inscription of Conducting the Qi, an unearthed cultural relic from the beginning of the Warring States Era (approximately 380 B.C.), talks about how to conduct the Qi as follows:

> When one conducts the Qi, the deeper one breathes, the more Qi one stores; the Qi extends downward, becomes fixed and consolidates. Then it germinates and grows upward and downward. One has to follow its natural course of circulation. If one does, one lives; and if not, one dies.

This indicates that there was a great deal of Qigong knowledge in existence at that time. There were two general interpretations of this passage. One was thinking of it as "Method of Real Qi Movement." The other was to consider it a "Method of Deep Breathing." But although it is truly the mind that leads the Qi, still the breathing and the movement of the Qi are connected. In the book *The Times of Slave System*, Guo Moruo pointed out:

> *It is one turn of deep breathing, inhale as much as you can, the Qi extends downward and steady; then breathing out, all the way up to the top. In this way, back and forth. If you follow this rule, you live; otherwise, you will die.*

2.3 QIGONG DURING THE XIANQIN DYNASTY (221–206 B.C.)

Lao Zi and Zhuang Zi, on behalf of the Dao Family, mentioned something about Qigong in their books. In the book *Lao Zi*, it was written:

> *Attain to the top of mind without thought. Keep calm. Calm down without thinking anything. Let your Qi seek to your lower Dantian. If you concentrate your Qi to pliability, you can get the flexibility as much as a baby does.*

These sayings not only reflect the philosopher's views, but also expound on the requirements of practicing Qigong. Zhuang Zi also talked about it. The idea is that when one breathes, one exhales old Qi and inhales new Qi, and one will live a long life. It is said that Peng Zhu of the Yin and Shang Era (approximately 1711–1066 B.C.) lived to be 800 years old. He was the first person who practiced Qigong in Chinese history and lived a long life.[3]

On behalf of the Ru Family, Kong Zi, in his book *Lun Yu*, said:

> *If you are a vegetarian, drink water, bend your arm instead of using a pillow when you sleep, and you will get joy from it.*

This is one kind of deep realization of experience. As to Yan Hui talking about sitting calmly, it has been described in the book *Zhuang Zi*, in which Yan Hui wrote:

> *I have been sitting and forgetting. I forget everything when I am sitting calmly." "What does that mean?" Zong Ni asked with amazement.*
> *Yan Hui answered: "Relax limbs, do not think of anything, let your mind go away from your body and become an object of the universe. This is sitting and forgetting.*

This is to say, you have forgotten the existence of your body when you sit for meditation. So Yan Hui's "sit and forget" in the book *Zhuang Zi* was the start for Chinese sitting meditation.

2.4 QIGONG DURING THE HAN DYNASTY (206 B.C.–220 A.D.)

Qigong developed further during the Han Dynasty. The "Guiding Chart for Breathing Exercises," as the name presently is given, was a work that consisted of different body postures and movements drawn on silk fabric. It was found at Tomb No. 3 of Mawang Dui (Ma Wang Mausoleum), Changsha City in 1973. From the same time, handed down in the ancient book from Zhanguo (380 B.C.) is an article called, "Do Not Eat, Just Do Breathing Exercise."

Because the son of Li Chong, prime minister of Changsha City, was buried under Tomb No. 3 of Mawang Dui in 168 B.C., the "Guide Picture" is a cultural relic, which is considered to belong to the early Han Dynasty.

In the later era of the Ma Wang Mausoleum in the Han Dynasty, Huainan Emperor Liu An inscribed a passage on practicing Qigong in his admonition of the spirit, "Huainan Zi":

> *In breathing exercises, one exhales the old air and inhales the new. Bears climb, birds fly, wild ducks swim, worms invigorate, hawks gaze and tigers look around—all these constitute the cultivation of the human nature.*

This passage has been called the "Game of Six Birds and Beasts" by people of later generations. The pity is that it did not offer any concrete methods for practicing Qigong.

Xun Yue also mentions in his work "Statements of Warnings" the use of guiding the Qi to help cure disease, and he stresses the importance of concentrating on the area beneath the navel. He says:

> *When one guides the stored Qi and circulates it inside the body, diseases can be cured. The area two inches below the navel is a pass where the Qi is stored and can be led to circulate through the whole body. . . That is why an important requirement is to guide and store the Qi in the pass.*

From all this we can see that Qigong had started to attract people's attention in ancient times—at least since the Han Dynasty—on a fairly wide scale. It had already been used to treat diseases, and the concept of storing Qi in the navel area had emerged.

Hua Tuo, a surgeon in the last years of East Han (approximately in the year 210 B.C.) compiled the "Game of Five Birds and Beasts," based on the theory that "running water is never stale and a door hinge never gets worm-eaten; constant movement creates Qi automatically," and the movements of the birds and beasts in the book *Huainanzi*. In a series of biographies in the *Book of Late Han*, Hua Tuo's account to his disciple Wu Pu on the "Game of Five Birds and Beasts," and the results Wu Pu got from practicing Qigong, reads:

> *Hua Tuo instructs and Wu Pu says 'A human body needs exercise but not excessive exercise. A body in movement eliminates stale breath and helps blood circulate. If one exercises, one doesn't get sick easily. This is just like the theory that a door-hinge never gets rusty.' Guiding Qi is something ancient immortals did all the time. 'Bears jump' and 'hawks gaze' are images of enhancing the movements of the joints of the human body—all this slows down the process of aging. I have a skill called the Game of Five Birds and Beasts: Number One is the tiger, Number Two the deer, Number Three the bear, Number Four the ape, and Number Five the bird. Exercise in guiding the Qi gets rid of disease and enhances the agility of the legs and feet. When one does not feel well, play the Game of the Five Birds and Beasts. One will sweat, feel pleasant and light, and have an appetite. If one persists in practicing in this manner, one will be able to see and hear clearly, and keep every one of one's teeth, even when one lives to be over ninety years old.*

The pity is that the concrete methods of practicing this set of "Game of the Five Birds and Beasts" has not been handed down over the centuries. However, the methods of practicing the Game have been sorted out and compiled by people of later generations.

2.5 QIGONG IN THE WEI, JIN, AND NAN BEI DYNASTIES (200–589 A.D.)

In "Dian Lun," Cao Pi (187–226 A.D.) said:

> *Gan Ling, Gan Shi, both of them know how to do breathing exercise; although they are old, their faces look like teenagers. In other words, if you know how to guide your Qi, you would always look younger. Later on, everybody who did Qigong exercises looked either like a bird or wolf, looking left and right, all around, breathing in new air and breathing out bad Qi.*

The *Book of the Hou Han* (Han Dynasty, circa 200 A.D.) says about Wang Zhen:

> *Although Wang Zhen is one hundred years old, he looks like he is only in his fifties. He can do breathing exercise with the navel and swallow the saliva in his mouth.*

Huang Pulong had discussed ancient Qigong with Cao Cao. In *Bei Ji Qian Jin Yao Fang*, Sun Simiao said:

> *Wei Wu tells Huang Pulong: "It's unbelievable that you are so healthy in your hundreds, your physical strength does not fail, your ears are very good, you have good eyesight. Your skin looks soft, smooth and full of joy. Would you tell me how can I get to that point?' Pulong answered, 'I heard about a Taoist priest, Kuai, Jing, who was strong at the age of 178. He would strike his teeth about twenty-seven times every morning until his mouth was full of saliva. Then he used it to wash his mouth and then swallowed the saliva. If you do it every day, you will be healthy."*

Bao Pu Zi, written by Ge Hong in the Jin Dynasty (265–420 A.D.) points out:

> *You can bend your torso forward, or lean your torso backward, or lean your torso to each side, or walk back and forth, or rest your body, or chant some words, or do breathing exercises. All of this is good for you.*

He also said:

> *When you know how to exhale and circulate the Qi, you will prolong your life. When you know how to extract and extend the Qi, you will slow down the process of getting old.*

At the same time, the word of "Three Dantian" came from *Pao Pu Zi*. "Dantian" is the name of a place in the human body. There are actually three of them, at upper, middle, and lower locations. The upper Dantian is located at a point between the eyebrows. The middle Dantian is between the nipples. Finally, the lower Dantian is located two inches below the navel.

It is said that the first reference to the term "Qigong" was by Xu Xun, in his book *Jing Ming Zong Jiao Lu* in the Jin Dynasty.

Tao Hongjing (451–536 A.D.) in the Nan Bei Dynasty was both a follower of Taoism and a doctor. In "Breathing and Treating Diseases," a section of his book *Ming Yi Bie Lu*, he talked not only about methods of breathing but also said:

> *All breathing exercises are inhale using the nose, exhale using the mouth. Guiding a little Qi breathing is called deep breathing. There is one way of inhaling the Qi, that is 'Xi'. There are six ways of exhaling the Qi: blowing, emitting, sighing, puffing out, heaving, and hissing. When you breathe, you exhale and inhale air. Exhalation has different functions. When you are cold, you blow out or emit warmth; when something is*

hot, you blow to drive the heat and you emit to eliminate the wind; you sigh to get rid of worries; you puff to enhance circulation of the Qi; you hiss to open up blockage; and you heave to release.

Before this time, all breathing exercises mainly concentrated on practicing inhalation. The emphasis on exhalation while doing breathing exercises started with Taoist practices. People later called it the 'Six-Word Rhymed Formula." The Formula can also apply to diseases of the five internal organs. The inscription says:

For heart disease, you blow and emit the Qi to drive away the cold and heat inside the body. For lung disease, you heave the Qi to reduce the swelling air in the lungs. For spleen disease, as there is air floating inside the body, you sigh out the Qi to relieve the itching, pain and stuffiness you feel. For liver disease, you puff out the Qi to get rid of the sour in the eyes and melancholy spirit.

Finally, this book refers often to Dong Gong, which is very popular now. This includes tooth bump (biting), mouth washing with your own saliva, wolf squat, hawk's gaze, lift the heel and bump the ground, pointing your toes back and forth, massaging your eyes, ears, and face, pushing up or raising your arms, and pushing your hands forward, among others.

2.6 QIGONG DURING THE SUI TANG AND WUDAI DYNASTIES (581–979 A.D.)

Ancient Qigong was very popular in the medical field during the Sui Tang Dynasty. Sun Simiao said in his *She Yang Zhen Zhong Fang*:

If your breathing is correct, you can prevent diseases; if your Qi is out of balance, you will get sick; if you are good at getting energy, you must know the methods of adjusting Qi; if you know how to adjust the Qi, you can prevent all diseases.

The truth is that breathing is very important to your health. On specifically how to do the exercise, he said:

The methods of adjusting Qi, between midnight to noon is life Qi; you can adjust the Qi. Between noon to midnight is die Qi; you cannot adjust the Qi. When you adjust the Qi, you should lie on your back, make the bed soft, make the pillow as high as your body, relax the entire body, four fingers grasp the thumb slightly, two hands five inches away from your legs, two feet five inches apart. Bite your teeth until your mouth is full of saliva, then swallow your saliva. Breathe in with your nose, breathe out through your mouth slowly. After taking a deep breath in, hold your breath. Count with your mind as many numbers as you can.

This was the method of breathing in. About breathing out, Sun Simiao wrote in *Six Words*:

People with cold diseases should Hu (emit) deeply thirty times. Hu gently ten times. The method is breathing out, breathing in through the nose, breathing out by the mouth. People with hot diseases should Chui (blow) deeply fifty times, Chui (blow) gently ten times. People with lung disease should Xu (heave) deeply thirty times and Xu (heave) gently ten times. People with liver diseases should He (puff out) deeply thirty times and He (puff out) gently ten times. People with spleen diseases should Xi (sigh) deeply thirty times and Xi (sigh) gently ten times. People with kidney diseases should Si (hiss) deeply thirty times and Si (hiss) gently ten times. It is important for someone to choose the treatment methods according to disease.

In the Sui Dynasty Zhi Yi, a founder of Buddhism, created a method called "Zhi Guan Fa." He talked about the body's breath and heart adjustment, which was a combination of gesture, breathing, and consciousness training methods. People who practiced martial arts adopted these methods.

Bai Juyi, the famous poet of the Tang Dynasty, always sat down quietly in his late years. In his *Jin Zuo Shi*, he said:

Sitting down quietly with eyes closed will adjust the breathing and be good for the skin. The first feeling is like having sweet wine, and the feeling that hibernating animals feel when they wake up, feeling the whole body relaxed and comfortable. I do not think of anything and forget where I am when I do breathing exercise.

He also said:

When I sit down quietly with my eyes closed in the midnight, I cannot hear my wife and children call me.

2.7 QIGONG DURING THE SONG, JIN, AND YUAN DYNASTIES (960–1368 A.D.)

At this time, ancient Qigong was combined with the inner Dan Shu of the Dao School. Also, Chinese medicine was blossoming, with many different schools emerging.

Sheng Ji Song Lu was a good book, combining both the theory and experience of medical science. It recorded some Qigong exercises related to guiding Qi and breath.

Zhang Rui, a professor during South Song Dynasty, said in his *Ji Feng Pu Ji Fang*:

> *Guiding the Qi by consciousness to where you don't feel comfortable, that would be treated well.*

This type of practice, which uses consciousness to guide the Qi, has been adopted by modern martial artists.

In *Lan Shi Mi Cang*, Li Dong Yuan pointed out how to cure diseases brought on by fatigue. A combination of sitting quietly and Chinese medicine is necessary.

The poet Lu You, during the Song Dynasty, was a practitioner of ancient Qigong. In his *Hao Shi Jing Ci*, he said:

> *Be calm down in your heart like the water in the lake without wind blowing, sit down and count your breath about thousands. . .*

Also, in his *Yong Shui* he said:

> *A host and a guest do consciousness facing each other with eyes closed at noon, both of them forgetting each other. The guest left after a while, but the host didn't know this until sunset, when he finished Qigong exercise.*

This was a kind of feeling of entering quietness for the Qigong practitioner. Related to the effect of practicing, he said in his *Xi Qian Lao Huai*:

> *Be in good health in your nineties, and get sharp eyes too.*

Ba Duan Jin, edited by an anonymous person, was a very popular method for people practicing Qigong between the North and South Song Dynasty.[4]

2.8 QIGONG DURING THE MING AND QING DYNASTIES (1368–1840 A.D.)

At this time, Qigong was mastered and used by people in the medical field. Wan Quan's *Ten Kinds of Wan Mi Zhai Medical Book* talked about quietly sitting. He wrote:

Sitting down and adjusting breathing is the key of stir Gong, never thinking of something else when doing this. The main method of practice quietly sitting is: Close your eyes; don't allow yourself to see something. Close your mouth; don't allow yourself to talk. Focus everything on your breathing.

As for breathing exercise, he said:

Adjusting breath should be adjusting true breath. The true breath is the fetus' breath. The fetus does not inhale and exhale in the womb, but the Qi is still circulating by itself. Doing exercise for long life, the breathing should be gentle and continuous, just as a fetus' breath in the womb.

Xu Chunpu, in the middle of the Ming Dynasty, edited *Ancient and Modern Medical Book*. It recorded many experiences about Qigong. He discussed both static and dynamic Qigong. There was also a self-massage set, which was encouraged for daily use. He said:

No matter if you have something to do or not, you should do the exercise at least once a day, doing self-massage more than thirty times at each joint from head to feet.

Shen Jiashu during the Qing Dynasty, emphasized in his *Yang Bing Yong Yan*:

Guiding breath is one hundred times better than medicine. You had better learn and know it.

In *Wei Shen Yao Shu*, Pan Weiru pointed out:

If you are not careful about your internal organs, muscles, and the weather change, it is easy to get sick. Ancient people cure themselves by acupuncture first, then guiding breath, massage, and so on. You would rather spend a short time doing some exercise every day to prevent disease than to get sick, and suffer the pain to see a doctor.

There was something related to Qigong in *Yun He Pian*, published at the end of the Qing Dynasty. *Secret Solution to a Problem of Shao Lin Martial Arts*, published at the beginning of the 20th Century, started with "Qigong Chan Wei." It said:

> *There were two ways to explain Qigong. One is "Yang Qi" and the other is "Lian Qi."*

Thereafter, the word "Qigong" was used broadly.

2.9 MODERN QIGONG (1840 A.D. TO PRESENT)

Qigong developed rapidly. It appeared in Jiang Wei-Qiao's *Yin Shi Zi Jing Zuo Fa*, Liu Guizhen's *Qigong Treatment Practice,* Fu Bao's *Jing Zuo Fa Jiang Yi,* Chen Qianming's *Jing De Xiu Yang Fa,* Hu Yaozhen's *Qigong,* Qin Zhongsan's *Lecture Sheets of Practical Qigong Treatment*, and other books.

The first professional Qigong treatment unit, Tangshan Qigong Hospital, was established at Tangshan, Hebei Province in 1955. It implemented some clinical observations, summarized the clinical practical materials, and popularized the way of "Inner Health Care Gong." It cured chronic intestinal and stomach diseases very well.

Through practice and research since 1958, many institutions prevented diseases by using Qigong. It got good results with chronic diseases such as ulcers, gastroptosis, high blood pressure, pulmonary tuberculosis, etc.

In respect to preventing disease, it started with the treatment of chronic diseases and developed to treatment of chronic hepatitis, excessive heartbeat, tuberculin (TB), pulmonary emphysema, high blood pressure, asthma, neurasthenia, diabetes mellitus, nephrosis, glaucoma, toxemias of pregnancy, metroptosis, chronic pelvic infection, etc. Qigong can also treat some acute diseases such as appendicitis, and can also help in some operations and anesthesia.

2.10 WILD GOOSE QIGONG

Wild Goose Qigong belongs to the Kunlun School, so it is also called Kunlun School Qigong. This school began in the Sichuan Province in China. The most famous practitioner of Wild Goose Qigong was Dao An, who spread it during the Jin Dynasty (265–420 A.D.). Because he was the most famous teacher of Wild Goose Qigong, he was crowned as its founder by later generations.

Later on, Wild Goose Qigong spread to northern China, and was kept by Wan Yi at Wutai Mountain. Emperor Qian Long, during the Qing Dynasty, promoted religion and established temples all over the country so that Wild Goose Qigong could be passed down to the present.

Yang Meijun was born at the end of the Qing Dynasty. When she was thirteen years old, she started to learn Wild Goose Qigong from her grandfather. By 1998 she was over 104 years old, and still practicing it everyday, living a very healthy life and using Qigong to treat patients in Beijing.

While Yang Meijun was visiting her son in the city of Wuhan in 1985, she was appointed an "honored professor" by the Wuhan Institute of Physical Education, and agreed to teach Wild Goose Qigong at the institute for two years.

Between 1985 and 1987, I was lucky to live next door to her. At that time, I was an instructor in the Department of Wushu (Chinese Martial Arts) and a graduate student of Wushu at the Wuhan Institute of Physical Education. I was also a founder of the Qigong Research Association at the institute, and was very interested in Qigong. I learned Wild Goose Qigong from Yang Meijun. This book is based on what I learned at that time.

CHAPTER THREE

The Effects of Qigong

Qigong is one of the traditional Chinese "Breathing Exercises," self-healing exercises welcomed by people of the world. It has a long history and a great variety of forms and routines. Practicing Qigong has an all-around effect on all the organs and systems of the human body. It is also an important way of strengthening one's fitness and preventing disease. It has a curative effect on high blood pressure (hypertension), neurasthenia, heart disease, ulcer disease (such as gastric ulcer, peptic ulcer, duodenal ulcer, etc.), tuberculosis, asthma (such as alveolar asthma, bronchitic asthma, infective asthma, etc.), chronic hepatitis, and other chronic diseases. In China, Qigong exercises combined with medicine have become an important method of treating some diseases in hospitals and clinical work.

In fact, it could be claimed that China was the first country to encourage its population to apply physical exercises to keep fit and prevent diseases. In 400 B.C., it was stated in *Huang Di Nei Jing, Su Wen (The Yellow Emperor's Classics of Internal Medicine)*, the oldest medical classics of China, that most diseases are caused by coldness or heat, and the best way to cure those diseases is through physical exercise. In addition, scientists in ancient China worked out a theory explaining why and how physical exercises strengthen fitness and cure diseases. Two thousand years ago (about 220 B.C.), a famous Chinese physician, Hua Tuo, developed the "Wu Qin Xi"—five animal play, imitating the movements of birds, bears, tigers, monkeys, and deer—as physical exercises for strengthening the body. He said that if a person moved very often, the "Guqi," meaning the ill gas (or sick Qi) in the body would be removed from the blood in the arteries and veins, and thus the blood would flow smoothly. In this way, a person would not get sick easily. He said, "This is somewhat like a door hinge which never gets rusty because it turns round all the time."

In recent years, along with the development of science and technology, the Chinese people are more and more interested in how to live better and get rid of diseases to prolong life. More and more people are turning to Qigong and searching for the relationship between Qigong practice and the avoidance of premature aging.

3.1 THE EFFECTS OF QIGONG EXERCISE ON THE CENTRAL NERVOUS SYSTEM

The central nervous system is the hub that regulates and controls the activities of all the systems and organs of the human body. Human beings adapt themselves to environments, and re-form environments through their activities. The activities of the nervous system enable the functions and activities of all the systems and organs in the body to be unified and work cohesively. Any kind of Qigong training that can strengthen the functioning of the central nervous system will have an excellent effect on protecting the health of the whole body. This is the real virtue of Qigong. Doing Qigong exercises, using the mind to control and lead the movements, will have good influences upon the central nervous system.

In addition, Qigong has a good medical effect on chronic diseases. The physiological mechanism of this is that, while practicing Qigong, most parts of the cortex are generally in a state of complete restraint (under control), except those concerned with central motor nerve and the second signal system, which are in the state of highly concentrated excitement.[5] This is because the excitement of the central motor nerve causes a negative change to the areas around it. As a result, the inhibition process is strengthened, and the dominant focus of excitation of chronic disease is inhibited. Therefore, the cells of the sick area can get positive rest. In this way, some of the symptoms ease off or disappear. Besides this, frequent engagement in Qigong exercise can improve the sensitivity of the nerve process and the stability of the sense of position.

3.2 THE EFFECTS OF QIGONG EXERCISE ON THE CARDIOVASCULAR SYSTEM

The effects of Qigong exercises on the cardiovascular system result from the controlled activities of the central nervous system. In terms of Qigong, when *Qingqi*, the clean gas in the body goes up, and *Zhuoqi*, the turbid gas comes down, abdominal pressure rises, and the veins in the abdominal cavity suffer pressure and carry the blood to the right atrium of the heart. Conversely, the blood is carried to the abdominal cavity when abdominal pressure comes down. Thus, not only is blood circulation increased, but a massage effect on the liver is produced by the movement of the abdominal muscles and diaphragm, thereby removing blood clots in the liver, improving its function, quickening and strengthening the process of metabolism, and ensuring stable blood pressure.

Doing Qigong can also strengthen the contraction of the heart muscles and increase the output capacity of every heartbeat. After doing Qigong exercises for a long time, the capacity of the heart is increased.[6] Therefore, the blood pumped out by the heart is increased, the utilization ratio of blood-oxygen in the body is improved, the elasticity of blood vessels is increased, and peripheral resistance is decreased. Consequently, the contracting of the heart is easier. Blood can be pumped farther by the heart's contraction but without great effort. All this will strengthen the functioning of the cardiovascular system, promoting physical fitness and stabilizing the blood pressure. Evidence clearly shows that a person who constantly exercises Qigong has a slow pulse rate when calm, and the blood pressure is lower than the normal value of someone the same age.[7] In people who practice Qigong, the pulse rate and systolic blood pressure rises less and the time for recovery is shorter than normal. This phenomenon is called "economic functioning." All of these are positive effects that Qigong has on the cardiovascular system.

The Research Group of the Chinese Gongfu Institute (comprised of myself and another Wushu Master, two medical doctors, and one research assistant from Northwestern University) has done research recording the number of heartbeats per minute for fifty people, resting ten minutes before practicing Qigong. The average number of heartbeats per minute is 75.1. The heartbeats are weak and fast. The number of heartbeats per minute decreases to 61 beats per minute after practicing twenty minutes of Qigong, the average decrease being 14.1. Ten people had heartbeats decrease to less than 53 beats per minute. The heartbeats are strengthened and slowed.

The heart beats about seventy times per minute. There are two kinds of nerves associated with the heart. One belongs to the sympathetic nerve, which strengthens and speeds up the heartbeat; the other belongs to the vagal (vice-sympathetic) nerve, which slows the heartbeat. Therefore, the heartbeat is slowed when you practice Qigong, reflected in the increased intensity of the heart vagal, and the decreased intensity in the sympathetic nerves of the heart.

We also have done research on high blood pressure in fifteen people who did relaxation Qigong exercises for twenty-five minutes. The blood pressure dropped from 156/99 mmHg to 135/81 mmHg after one year of Qigong exercise. The systolic blood pressure dropped 21 mmHg and the diastolic pressure dropped 18 mmHg.

Cholesterol is an important blood fat. It can be obtained by eating animal fats (such as eggs, cheese, cream, liver, pork, beef, etc.). Increased cholesterol values correlate with a tendency towards atherosclerosis. Values of 200 mg or less are associated with a lower risk of heart attacks and strokes. The desirable range for people under forty is less than 200 mg; for those over forty, the desirable range is 220–240 mg.

People with a family history of heart attacks or stroke should pay special attention to cholesterol so they can prevent these conditions. One way to prevent high cholesterol is not to eat too much meat or junk food. Another way, which is the best way, is to take Qigong or Taiji exercise at least twice a week.

3.3 THE EFFECTS OF QIGONG EXERCISES ON THE METABOLIC SYSTEM (METABOLISM)

Improving metabolism is an important function of Qigong for health. Many diseases are associated with poor metabolism. Practicing Qigong can improve the metabolic activity of tissue cells, especially the ability of anabolic metabolism and, consequently, increase their ability to resist degeneration, sclerosis, and death. This shows that practice of Qigong can prolong one's life.

Experiments with older persons have also shown that the content of cholesterol in blood decreased after doing Qigong exercises for ten minutes. This is especially true of patients with higher cholesterol.

3.4 THE EFFECTS OF QIGONG EXERCISES ON THE DIGESTIVE SYSTEM

As the capability of the nervous system is improved, the functional activities of other systems will also be improved. This can prevent and treat some afflictions of the digestive system, which result from functional disturbances of the nervous system. In addition, the respiratory movement, which provides mechanical stimuli to the gastrointestinal tract, can also improve the blood circulation of the alimentary tract, so that digestion is promoted and constipation is prevented. This is very important.

3.5 THE EFFECTS OF QIGONG EXERCISES ON THE RESPIRATORY SYSTEM

We have done research on the number of breaths per minute for thirty people. Their ages were between thirty-five and fifty-five. They practiced ten Qigong movements for twenty minutes in each class, twice a week for one year. The average number of breaths per minute was fourteen before practicing Qigong. The average decreases to 4.3 times per minute after practicing twenty minutes of Qigong. There were twelve people whose breaths per minute decreased to less than four.

Frequency of breathing is the number of breaths (inhale and exhale) per minute. Generally, the number of breaths per minute for adults is about seventeen. There is an obvious decrease in the number of breaths per minute when you do Qigong exercise, improving the function of the respiratory system, and reflecting that the cerebral cortex is at a subdued state. This is a good method of self-healing for people who have pneumonia, bronchitis, asthma, and tuberculosis.

3.6 THE EFFECTS OF QIGONG ON CANCER AND AIDS

There have been several cases of my students suffering from cancer who have apparently been cured, and others whose condition has seemed to be stabilized or improved with Qigong. Examples include four students with breast cancer. One of them had cancer cells already present in the lymph of her armpit. She started practicing Qigong after an operation to remove the breast and lymph. She practiced Qigong every day except for the days she went for chemotherapy. The doctor let her visit the chiropractor, but she practiced Qigong instead. Now, three years later, she can do everything. The Qigong provided an excellent complement to her modern medical treatments. She even started a full-time job a few months ago.

One of my other students had skin cancer on her calf. She had had surgery three times and almost all of the muscle of her calf was gone. "You will never have feeling in your lower calf," her doctor said. "It was true. The first month after surgery, I didn't feel cold, heat, pain, or sense of touch—only numbness," said the student. "I have feeling now," she told me after practicing Qigong for three months. If you watch her walk and practice Qigong, you would never believe that she had skin cancer on her calf.

One of my students with cancer said, "Last year I was diagnosed with a malignant brain tumor. Luckily they were able to remove it, and now, while going through radiation and chemotherapy, I am studying Qigong with Master Zhang, which I find gives me more energy and better concentration so I can focus on my sense of wellness instead of the illness."

I had a student who was a famous ballet dancer in the early 1980s. He came to my school for private lessons to learn Qigong. He used his fingers and knuckles or the corners of the tables and walls to press against his back in the area of his kidneys during the class. "Why do you do this?" I asked. "It can relieve a little bit of pain, which I have had more than ten years," he said. I never saw him do this again after he learned Qigong with me for three months. "You did not press your kidneys," I said to him one day. He said, "I do not have that pain anymore." Then he attended my Taiji group lessons one year later and continued to practice Taiji more than two years with the same group. "I am glad that I came to you to learn Qigong and Taiji. I am feeling great. My life is replenished with wellness. I have never had this kind of nice feeling the past fifteen years. I hope I can return to my Qigong and Taiji classes again. Unfortunately, I do not have any power. It is time to go now." He was calling me from the hospital. He passed away a few days later because he had had AIDS for many years.

3.7 THE EFFECTS OF QIGONG ON DISPOSITION

Many students report that practicing Qigong has had a good effect on their dispositions. For example, they are less easily upset by daily events that would previously have made them angry. Qigong has the effect of making people feel calm and they feel more able to handle stressful situations.

I forget a bad day, I am full of energy, and feel more relaxed. I feel great," *one of my students told me after class. "What are you talking about?" I asked* *him. He said, "I came to class after a very difficult workday. I had been* *angry in meetings with people who had tried to steal one of my clients from* *me and then had lied about it. I felt tense, nervous, and tired. But now,* *after class, I am calmer and not so worried about what has happened at* *work. I feel relaxed and great."*

CHAPTER FOUR

Training Method of Wild Goose Qigong

THE PRE-64 FORM

FORM 1 Starting Form

Stand upright naturally, feet parallel and shoulder-width apart. Let your arms hang naturally by the side of your thighs. Close your mouth slightly with the tip of the tongue touching the root of the teeth. Look ahead (Figure 1-1).

Notes: Keep your head and neck erect. Relax your shoulders and hips. Breathe naturally through your nose. Meditate for a few moments to gain concentration. Calmly guide your movements.

Effects: Relieves tension in the neck, shoulders and arms, and focuses your thoughts at your lower Dantian.

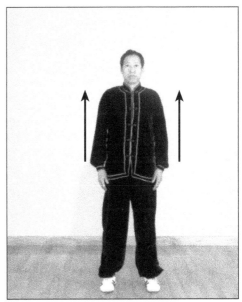

Figure 1-1

FORM 2 Spread the Wings

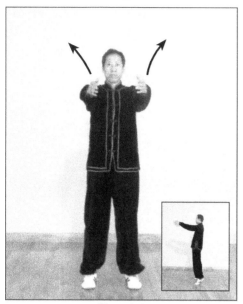

Figure 2-1

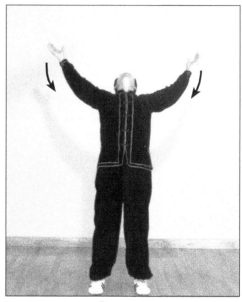

Figure 2-2

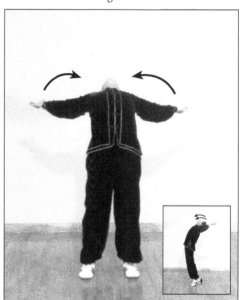

Figure 2-3

1. Keeping your arms shoulder-width apart, raise them to shoulder level with your palms facing each other. At the same time, lift your heels from the floor. Look straight ahead (Figure 2-1).

2. Continue the last movement without stopping. Spread your arms out with the palms up. Slightly bend your knees and keep your heels off the floor. Bend your torso backward as far as you can. Look toward the sky (Figures 2-2, 2-3).

Notes: Maintain a slow, steady pace while raising your arms and throughout your practice. The extent to which you stretch, bend your back, or lift your heels is an individual matter. Go only as far as is comfortable. With practice, your flexibility will improve.

Effects: Stretches your muscles, strengthens your lungs and keeps the vertebral column straight.

FORM 3 Close the Wings

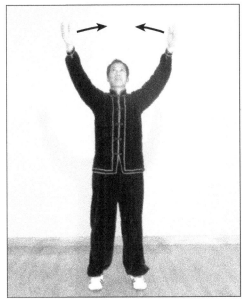

Figure 3-1

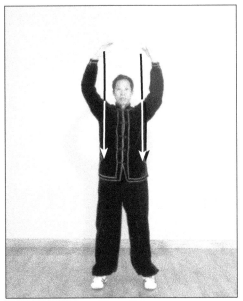

Figure 3-2

1. Bending your elbows slightly, turn your arms in while they are still raised upward, forward over your head, thumbs pointing toward each other with palms down. At the same time, your heels touch the floor. Keep your torso upright. Look ahead (Figures 3-1, 3-2).

2. Continue the last movement without stopping, and lower your palms slowly to both sides of the lower Dantian, with your hands about one to two inches apart, thumbs pointing toward each other. Leave about two inches between your palms and abdomen. Bend your elbows slightly. Look ahead (Figure 3-3).

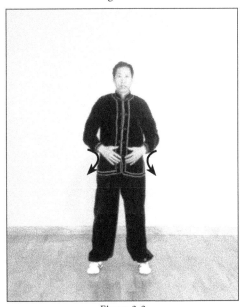

Figure 3-3

Notes: Relax your whole body naturally. Keep your mind focused at the lower Dantian.

Effects: Helps relieve nervousness, dizziness, and stomach disorders. Increases circulation.

FORM 4 Fold Nest

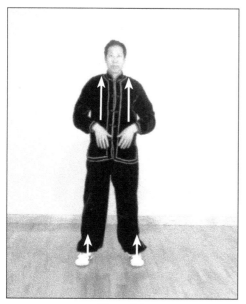

Figure 4-1

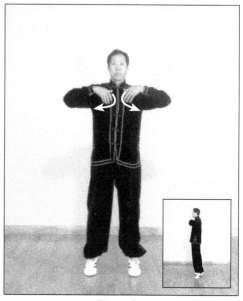

Figure 4-2

1. Bend your elbows and raise both hands slowly to chest level with your palms facing your chest. At the same time, lift your heels off the floor (Figures 4-1, 4-2).

2. Then turn your arms in until your palms are facing forward, fingers pointing toward each other. Look ahead (Figure 4-3).

3. Continue the last movement and push your palms forward until your arms are straight, palms facing forward, thumbs pointing down (Figure 4-4).

4. Spread your arms backward to both sides, keeping them straight (Figure 4-5). Then bend your arms toward your back until your thumbnails or the back of each hand touches

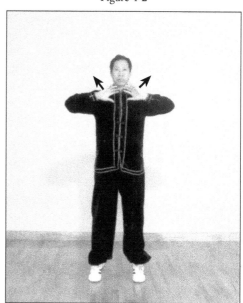

Figure 4-3

acupressure point B18 at both sides of your spine (Figure 4-6). Continuing the last movement without stopping, press your thumbnails down past B19, B20, B21, and B22 in order. Look ahead (Figure 4-7).

Notes: Keep your balance. Relax your shoulders.

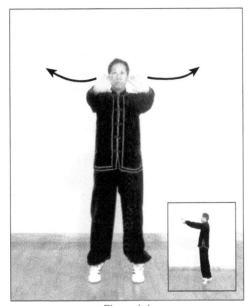

Figure 4-4

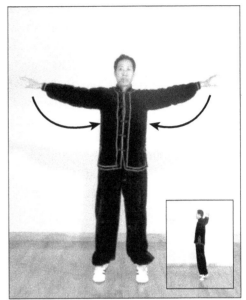

Figure 4-5

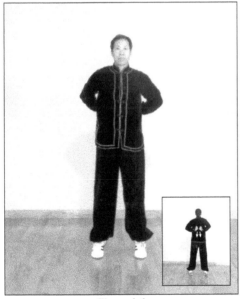

Figure 4-6

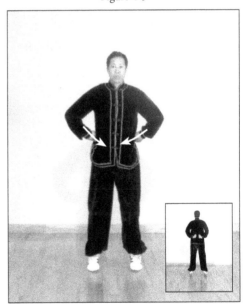

Figure 4-7

Effects: This movement is good for liver disease, eye disease, poor digestion, anemia, stomach disease, back pain, kidney disease, neurasthenia, irregular menstruation, and so on.

FORM 5 Shake Wings

Swing your arms forward with elbows bent about ninety degrees. Press B52, G26, and S25 with your thumb and forefinger in order, fingers pointing forward and palms up. At the same time, your heels touch the floor. Look ahead (Figure 5-1).

Notes: Coordinate the movement of your arms and feet.

Effects: This is good for kidney deficiency. It helps relieve pain in the waist and legs, and helps correct stomach disorders.

FORM 6 Fold Nest

Repeat steps #1 through #4 of Form 4, Fold Nest (see Figures 4-1, 4-2, 4-3, 4-4, 4-5, 4-6, and 4-7).

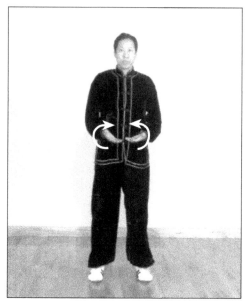

Figure 5-1

FORM 7 Shake Wings

Repeat Form 5, Shake Wings (see Figure 5-1).

FORM 8 Raising Wings

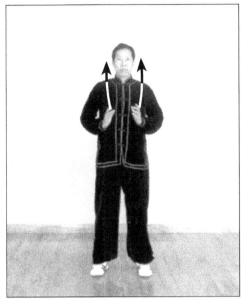

Figure 8-1

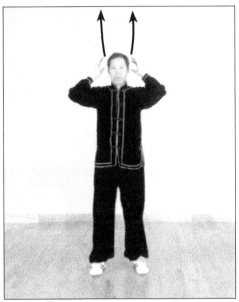

Figure 8-2

Keep standing with your feet shoulder-width apart.

1. Turn your arms in with palms facing each other, fingers pointing up (Figure 8-1).

2. Continuing the last movement without stopping, raise your arms slowly until they are straight, keeping your shoulders relaxed and palms facing each other, shoulder-width apart. Look at your palms (Figures 8-2, 8-3).

Notes: Relax your shoulders as you raise your arms.

Effects: Helps relieve tennis elbow and stiffness in the neck, shoulders, and waist.

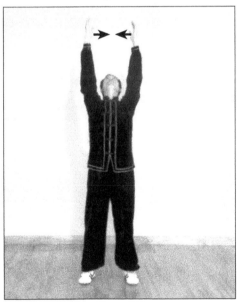

Figure 8-3

FORM 9 Cross Wings

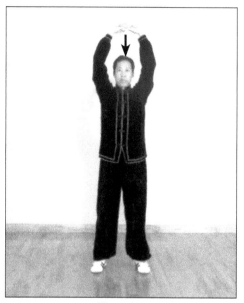 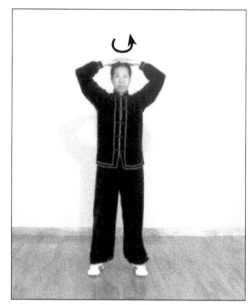

Figure 9-1   Figure 9-2

Keep your feet in the same position as above. Interlock your fingers above your head naturally while straightening your neck (Figure 9-1), and then press down until your palms touch your head. Look ahead (Figure 9-2).

Notes: Coordinate the movements of your hands and head.

Effects: This helps lower high blood pressure, relieve headaches, dizziness, and anal prolapse, and helps relieve and prevent the effects of stroke.

FORM 10 Push Wings Upward

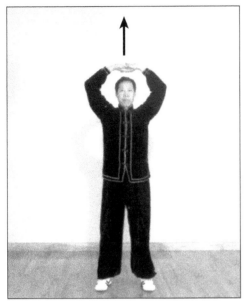 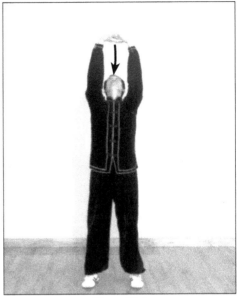

Figure 10-1   Figure 10-2

Keeping your fingers interlocked, rotate your arms until your palms face up (Figure 10-1). Then push up with your palms until your arms are straight. At the same time, look at your hands. Keep your feet in the same position as above with your legs straight (Figure 10-2).

Notes: Straighten your waist and arms; relax your shoulders.

Effects: Helps keep the vertebral column straight and strengthens the neck, shoulder joints, and waist.

FORM 11 Crossed Wings Touch the Ground (Center, Left, Right)

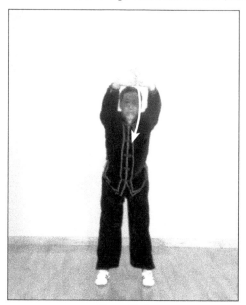
Figure 11-1

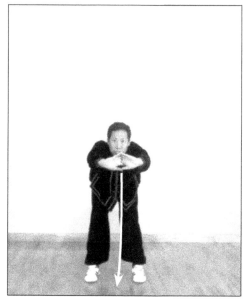
Figure 11-2

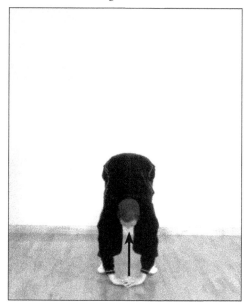
Figure 11-3

1. While keeping your legs and backbone straight, bend your torso forward and press down with your palms, keeping your fingers interlocked. Touch the floor with your palms for three seconds. Look ahead and down about five feet in front of you (Figures 11-1, 11-2, 11-3).

2. Straighten your torso without moving your feet. At the same time, raise your hands with your arms turned out, palms in. Look ahead (Figures 11-4, 11-5).

3. Keep your legs straight and turn your torso to the left side. Turn your arms in until your palms face down (Figure 11-6). Press down with interlocked fingers until your palms touch the floor for three seconds. Look down and to the left about five feet away (Figure 11-7).

4. Raise your torso and turn right 180 degrees. Repeat #2 above (Figures 11-8, 11-9, 11-10).

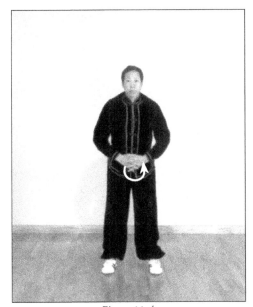

Figure 11-4

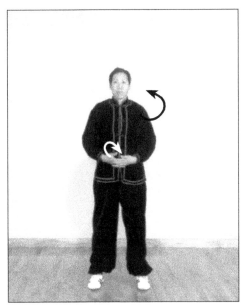

Figure 11-5

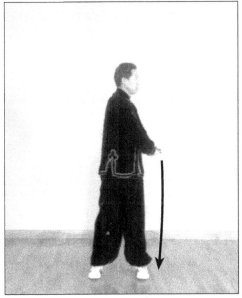

Figure 11-6

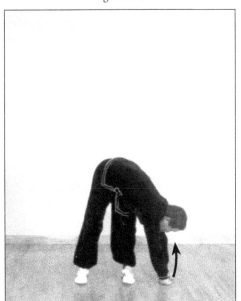

Figure 11-7

5. Repeat #3 above, pressing your palms to the right side (Figure 11-11).

Notes: Keep your legs and backbone straight. How low you press down with interlocked fingers depends on you. Go only as far as you feel comfortable.

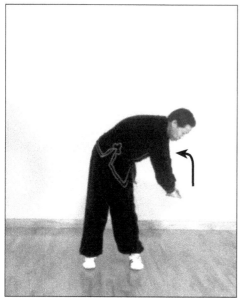

Figure 11-8

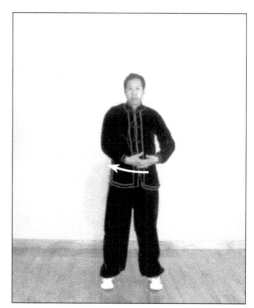

Figure 11-9

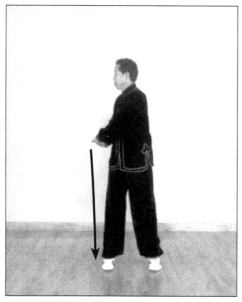

Figure 11-10

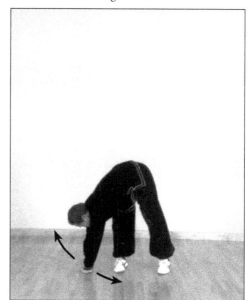

Figure 11-11

Effects: Stretches the tendons and muscles of the shoulders, legs, and waist. Relieves stiffness in shoulders, waist, and legs. Increases circulation.

FORM 12 Cross Wings

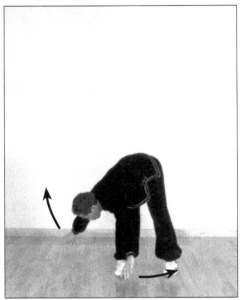

Figure 12-1

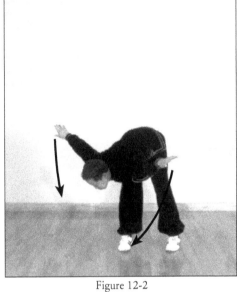

Figure 12-2

1. Raise your torso about forty-five degrees while turning back to the center. Spread both arms out, the left arm at forty-five degrees between front and left, the right arm at forty-five degrees between back and right. Fingers point outward, palms face down. Bend your knees slightly (Figures 12-1, 12-2).

2. Raise your torso and lower both hands. Meanwhile, turn your arms out until your palms face up, and then cross your arms in front of your right chest, left arm on the outside. Keep your feet in the same position as above (Figures 12-3, 12-4).

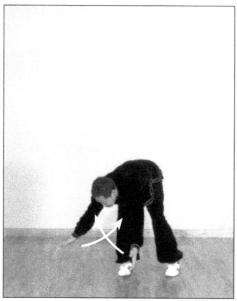

Figure 12-3

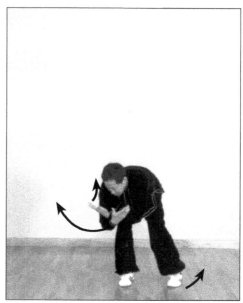

Figure 12-4

Notes: Coordinate crossing your arms with raising your torso.

Effect: Strengthens muscles of the legs and waist and prevents and relieves pain in the lower back and knees.

FORM 13 Recover Air

1. Bend your right leg without moving your right foot. Your left foot turns out ninety degrees with the heel touching the floor. Keeping your left foot flat on the floor, shift your weight onto your right leg to form a left empty stance. At the same time, your left hand forms a claw (five fingers touching each other at their tips) and raises until your fingers point to S12 on the left side. Relax your shoulders naturally. Your right hand and arm arc downward, back and upward to head level, turning your arm out until your palm faces up. Look at your right hand (Figures 13-1, 13-2).

2. Bend your torso to the left side. At the same time, the right hand arcs up, leftward, and down to the left toes. Raise the toes of your left foot, keeping your heel on the floor. Bend your right knee and keep your left knee straight. Keep your weight on your right foot. Look at your right hand (Figures 13-3, 13-4).

Notes: Coordinate bending your torso with pulling back your left toes.

Effects: Strengthens and stretches muscles. Persevere in the exercise. It is good for stomach disorders, distended chest, and pains in the waist.

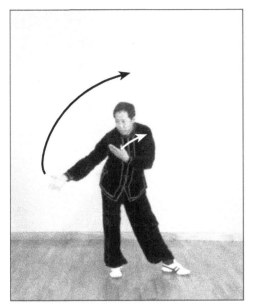

Figure 13-1

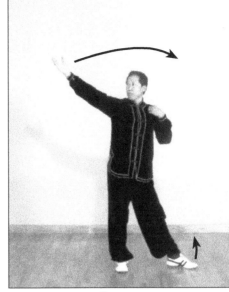

Figure 13-2

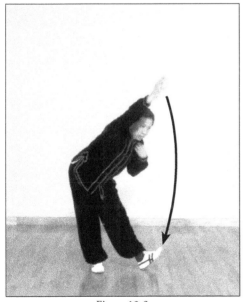

Figure 13-3

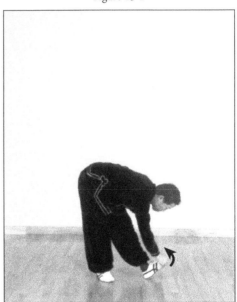

Figure 13-4

FORM 14 Spread Left Foot (Three Times)

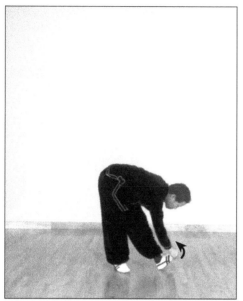
Figure 14-1

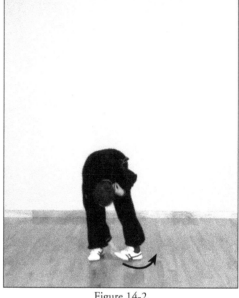
Figure 14-2

Press points Liv2 and Liv3 with your right thumb, and the web between your right thumb and forefinger facing the SP1 point, the other fingers resting under your toes. Push your left foot to the left about forty-five degrees (Figure 14-1), and then pull it back to the right about 135 degrees with your right hand (Figure 14-2).

Repeat turning your foot a total of three times back and forth. At the same time, twist your torso naturally without moving your right foot.

Notes: Coordinate pushing your toes with turning your body.

Effects: Relieves headache, dizziness, insomnia, stomachache, fever, and bleeding of the uterus. Strengthens the legs while also increasing the pliability and toughness of the muscles.

FORM 15 Push Air

Turn your torso to the right about ninety degrees, keeping your waist and hips relaxed. Turn your left foot to the right until your toes point forward, and then keep your foot flat on the floor. At the same time, shift your weight on both feet. Slowly push your right hand forward from the left side to the right side, palm down, fingers pointing forward. Your left hand doesn't move. Look at your right hand (Figures 15-1, 15-2, 15-3, 15-4).

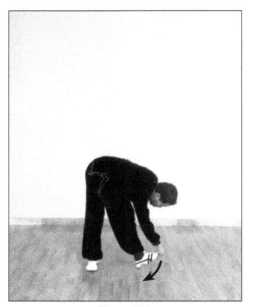
Figure 15-1

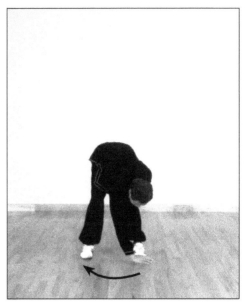
Figure 15-2

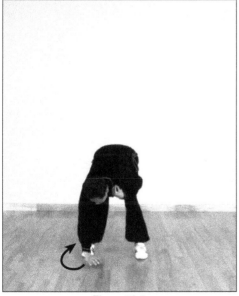
Figure 15-3

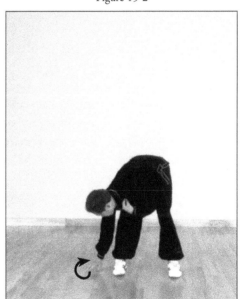
Figure 15-4

Notes: Coordinate turning your torso with pushing your right hand to the right. Concentrate on point P8.

Effects: Helps remove bad Qi from the body. Strengthens waist muscles.

FORM 16 Drag in Air

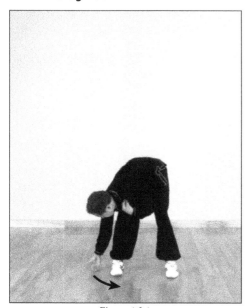
Figure 16-1

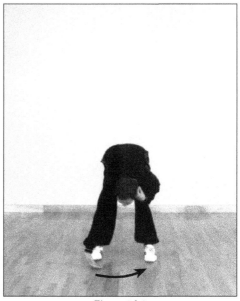
Figure 16-2

Turn your right arm out until the palm faces up, fingers pointing to the left and bending your arm slightly. Then turn your torso to the left. At the same time, your right hand drags in air to the left. Your left hand and both feet remain unchanged. Look at your right hand (Figures 16-1, 16-2, 16-3).

Notes: Coordinate dragging air with turning your torso.

Effects: Helps pull energy from the earth.

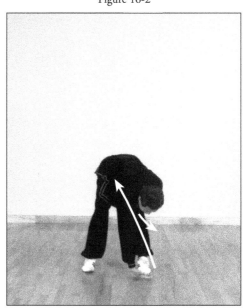
Figure 16-3

FORM 17 Turn Body and Recover Air

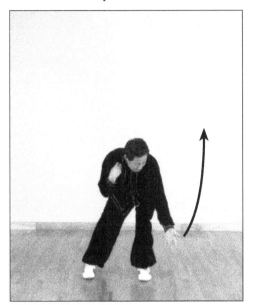

Figure 17-1

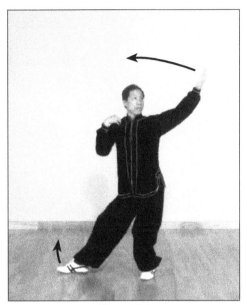

Figure 17-2

Raise your torso and turn ninety degrees to the right while the left claw hand opens and your right foot turns out ninety degrees. Meanwhile, your left hand arcs downward, back, and upward to about head level, turning your arm out until your palm faces up. At the same time, your right hand forms a claw, five fingers touching each other at their tips, and then rises until your fingers point to S12 on the right side when you turn right (Figures 17-1, 17-2).

Repeat step #2 of Form 13, reversing right and left (Figure 17-3).

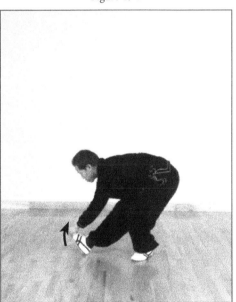

Figure 17-3

FORM 18 Spread Right Foot (Three Times)

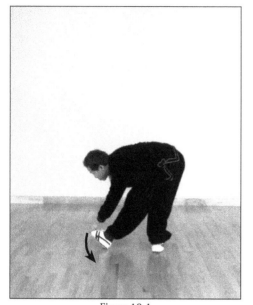

Figure 18-1

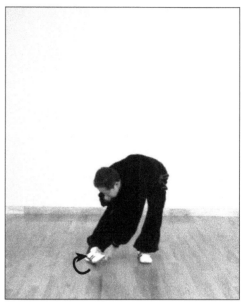

Figure 18-2

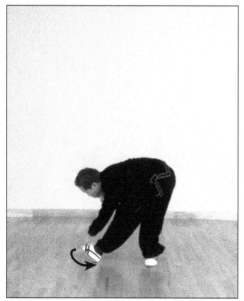

Figure 19-1

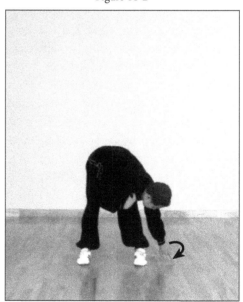

Figure 19-2

Repeat Form 14, reversing right and left (Figures 18-1, 18-2).

FORM 19 Push Air

Repeat Form 15, reversing right and left (Figure 19-1, 19-2).

FORM 20 Drag in Air (Left)

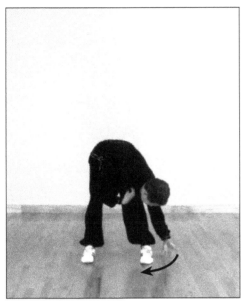

Figure 20-1

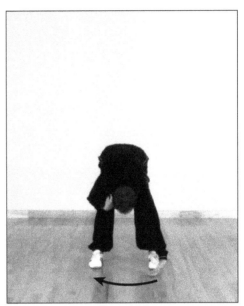

Figure 20-2

Repeat Form 16, reversing right and left (Figures 20-1, 20-2, 20-3).

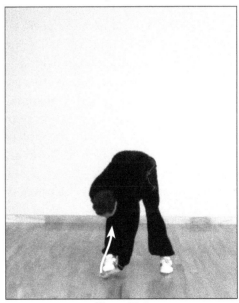

Figure 20-3

FORM 21 Twirling Wings

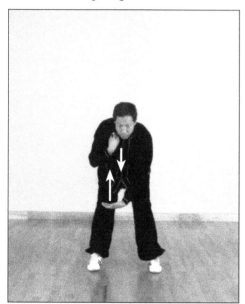

Figure 21-1

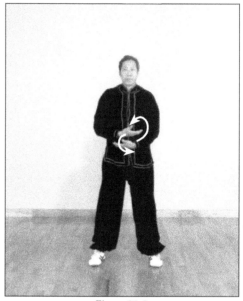

Figure 21-2

1. Raise your torso and return to the center, facing front. Turn your right foot in ninety degrees so that both feet are parallel, pointing forward and shoulder-width apart. At the same time, raise your left hand in front of your abdomen with your palm up, fingers pointing to the right. Your right hand goes down to above the left hand, about two inches apart, palm up and fingers pointing to the left. Look at your left hand (Figures 21-1, 21-2).

2. Bend both knees slightly. Your right hand circles counter-clockwise around your left hand. At the same time, your left hand circles clockwise around the right hand. Both hands make their circles around each other

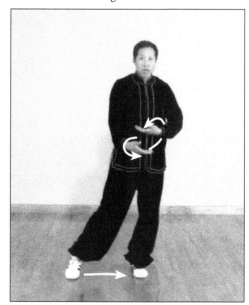

Figure 21-3

until the right hand is at the bottom. Both palms face up, five inches apart. Points P6 and TE5 of both hands should face each other. At the same time, shift your weight to your left foot and draw your right foot next to the left. Look at both hands (Figures 21-3, 21-4, 21-5).

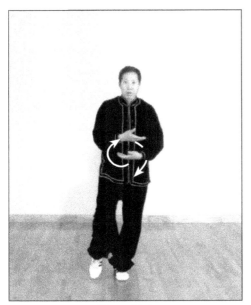

Figure 21-4

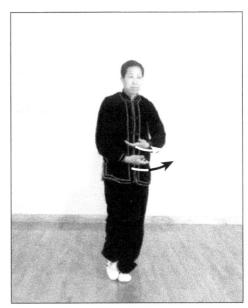

Figure 21-5

Notes: Sway your torso and arms naturally. Waist leads shoulders, shoulders lead arms, and arms lead hands when twirling wings.

Effects: This not only helps to prevent waist pain, back pain, chest pain, rib pain, headache, ringing ears, colds and fever, but also treats all of these conditions.

FORM 22 Wave Wings Like Clouds (Right, Left, Right)

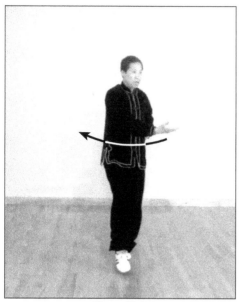

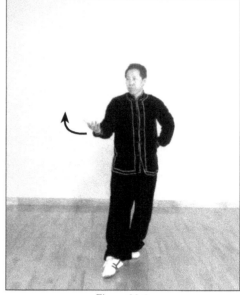

Figure 22-1   Figure 22-2

1. Wave Right Wing Like Clouds

(a.) Turn your torso to the left. At the same time, move your left hand to the left side at waist level with your palm upward. Then move your left hand back until point L14 of the left hand touches the left point B23 of the left waist (Figure 22-1) with the palm upwards at waist level.

(b.) Step forward with your right foot, small toe touching the floor first and bending your right knee slightly. At the same time, move your right hand to the right front with your palm upward at waist level. Bend your arm slightly. Look between center and right (Figure 22-2).

Notes: Coordinate shifting your weight with moving your left hand. Coordinate stepping with your right foot with moving your right hand.

Effects: This helps prevent and treat headache, toothache, tonsillitis, kidney disease, throat disease, injury to muscles of waist and arms, neurasthenia, and irregular menstruation.

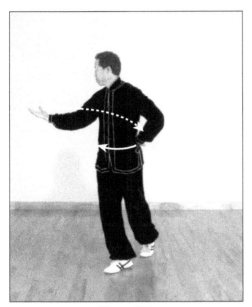

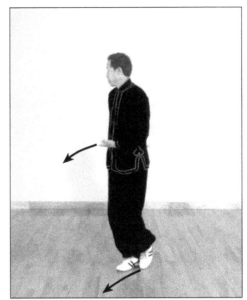

Figure 22-3   Figure 22-4

2. Wave Left Wing Like Clouds

(a.) Turn your torso to the right about forty-five degrees. While shifting your weight to the right foot, bring your left foot next to your right foot, move your left hand to the right side and turn your arm in. Then move your right hand backward until the point L14 of the right hand touches the point B23 of the right waist. At the same time, point L14 of your left hand presses B23, B52, G26, SP15, S25, and K16 points in order. Then turn your arm out until your palm faces upward and fingers are pointing to the right (Figures 22-3, 22-4).

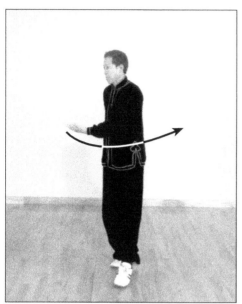

Figure 22-5

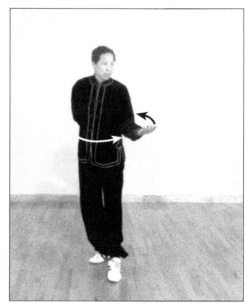

Figure 22-6

(b.) Step forward with your left foot, little toe touching the floor first and bending your left knee slightly. At the same time, move your left hand to the left front at waist level, palm upward. Look between left and center (Figures 22-5, 22-6).

Notes: Coordinate shifting your weight with moving your right hand. Follow the left foot with the left hand. Pressing the points should be coordinated with moving your left foot.

Effects: This can prevent and treat the same diseases as above, such as kidney disease, back pain, leg pain, stomach disorders, and so on.

3. Wave Right Wing Like Clouds

Repeat Wave Left Hand Like Clouds, reversing left and right (see Figures. 22-1, 22-2).

FORM 23 Twist Waist

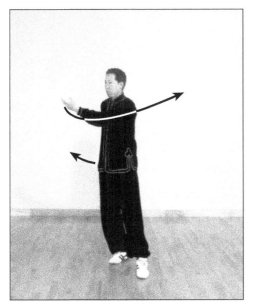

Figure 23-1

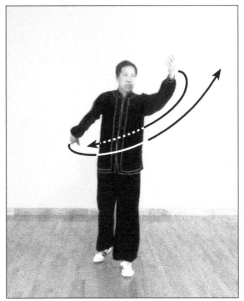

Figure 23-2

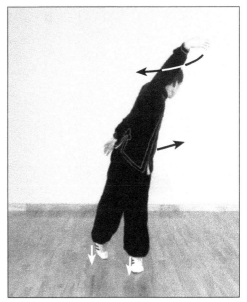

Figure 23-3

1. Repeat Form 22, #2a (see Figure 22-3).

2. Repeat Form 22, #2b, but your left hand is at shoulder level (Figure 23-1).

3. Shift your weight forward on your left foot with both legs straight and both heels off the floor. Twist your waist to the left about ninety degrees. At the same time, wave your left arm to the left, downward, and backward until your left palm faces G30. Wave your right hand to the left with your arm straight until your palm faces your right temple. Look at your left hand (Figures 23-2, 23-3).

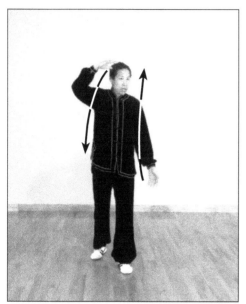

Figure 23-4

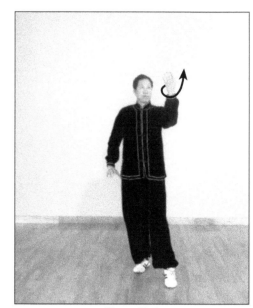

Figure 23-5

4. Shift your weight back quickly on your right foot with your left toes on the floor, forming a left empty stance. Turn your torso back to the center. At the same time, swing your right hand to the right side at waist level, fingers pointing forward with the palm downward. Your left arm scoops forward and up until your palm faces GV24.5. Look at your left palm (Figures 23-4, 23-5).

Notes: Shifting your weight coordinates with waving your arms.

Effects: Prevents and relieves backache. Helps to strengthen muscles in the back.

FORM 24 Lower Wing to Recover Air

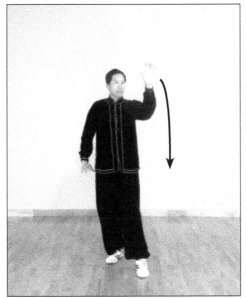

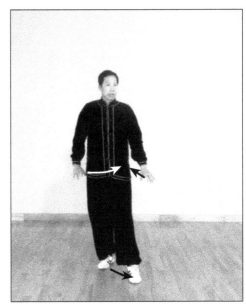

Figure 24-1   Figure 24-2

Turn your left arm inward until the palm faces forward. Then lower your left hand to the side of your left leg, palm facing backward, fingers pointing down. Look straight ahead (Figures 24-1, 24-2).

Notes: Lower your left arm naturally and keep the movements at the same speed.

Effects: Relieves stiffness in arms, wrists, and fingers.

FORM 25 Spread the Single Wing

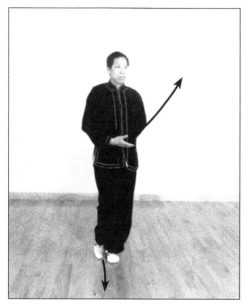
Figure 25-1

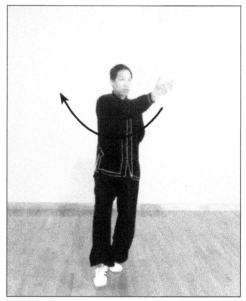
Figure 25-2

1. Repeat "Wave Right Wing Like Clouds," Form 22, #1a (Figures 25-1, 25-2).

2. Repeat "Wave Right Wing Like Clouds," Form 22, #1b, but your right hand is at eye level (Figure 25-3).

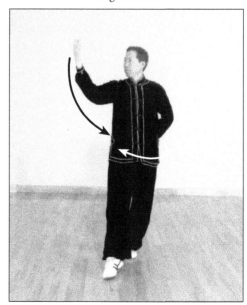
Figure 25-3

FORM 26 Fold Up Wings with "T" Step

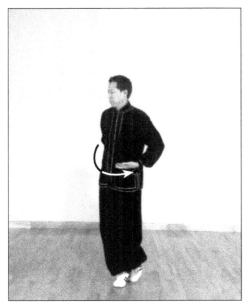 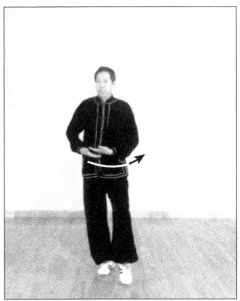

| Figure 26-1 | Figure 27-1 |

Repeat "Wave Left Wing Like Clouds," Form 22, #2a (Figure 26-1).

FORM 27 Encircle (Wind Hand Around) Head and Pass Ears

1. Step forward with your left foot, small toe touching the floor first. Point L14 of your right hand presses points B23, B52, G26, SP15, and K16 in order. Then turn your right arm out until your palm faces the back of your left hand (Wailaogong Point) as your torso turns right forty-five degrees (Figure 27-1).

2. With your right hand, press each point of the Sanjiao channel of hand-shaoyang in order from your left hand to your left shoulder. Then raise your right hand until the palm faces your left ear (Figures 27-2, 27-3, 27-4).

3. Then your right hand passes points behind the neck, GV16, GV15, B10, G12, until your palm faces your right ear. Look straight ahead (Figure 27-5).

Notes: Relax your shoulders and arms when winding your hand around your head and passing your ears.

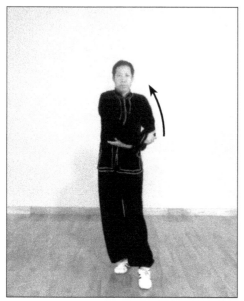

Figure 27-2

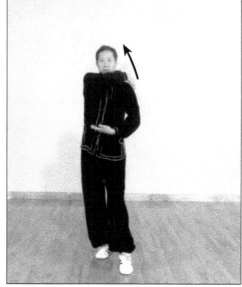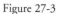

Figure 27-3

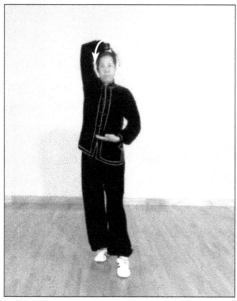

Figure 27-4

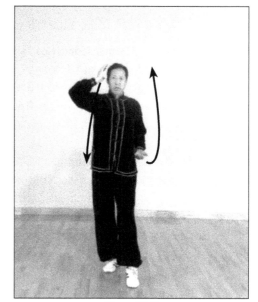

Figure 27-5

Effects: This movement helps prevent and treat pain in the shoulders, arms, elbows, diseases of the ears and eyes, neck disease, headache, and high blood pressure. It also has good effects on the fitness of the mind, promotes the brain to think, cleans away heat, and brightens the eyes, as well as invigorates the circulation of the blood, and so on.

FORM 28 Press Downward

Keep your feet in the same position as above. Your right palm presses down by your right hip bone, fingers pointing forward and separated. At the same time, raise your left hand forward to shoulder level with elbow bent slightly, palm facing up and slightly inward. Look at your left hand (Figure 28-1).

Notes: Coordinate pressing down with your right hand and lifting your left hand.

Effects: Pressing down with the right hand removes sick energy from the right hand and foot. Lifting the left hand draws energy from the left hand and foot. Thus, it regulates the balance of Yin and Yang to maintain health.

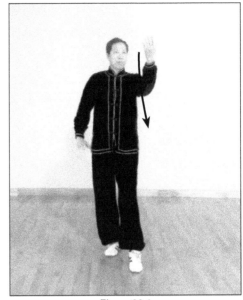

Figure 28-1

FORM 29 Lifting Wing

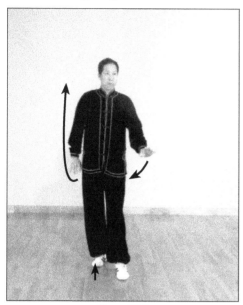
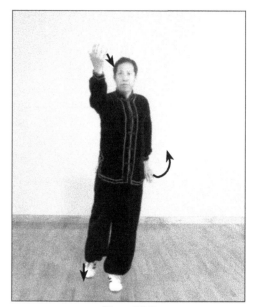

Figure 29-1   Figure 29-2

Shift your weight slowly onto your left foot, right heel off the floor, with both legs straight. At the same time, turn your right arm out until the palm faces upward. Then bring your hand forward, upward in a curve to shoulder level, fingers pointing forward. Bend your arm slightly. Turn your left arm in until your palm faces down. Then press your left palm down naturally to the left side of your hip, fingers pointing to the floor. Look at your right hand (Figures 29-1, 29-2).

Notes: Lifting your right hand and lowering your left hand should be coordinated with shifting your weight to your left foot.

Effects: Lifting your right hand draws energy from the earth and heaven through your right hand and right foot. Lowering your left hand removes sick energy from your left hand and left foot. Therefore, this regulates the balance of Yin and Yang and keeps you fit.

FORM 30 Recover Air

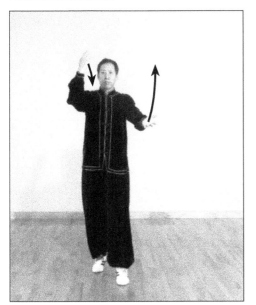

Figure 30-1

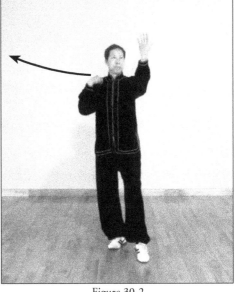

Figure 30-2

Quickly shift your weight to your right foot, right heel touching the floor and left toes touching the floor. Bend both knees slightly. At the same time, with all five fingertips touching one another, quickly bend your right forearm inward until your fingertips touch the S12 point. Your right elbow points between center and right. Meanwhile, turn your left arm in until your palm faces forward. Then bring your left hand forward and up in a curve to head level, palm facing your forehead. There should be about one hundred degrees between your forearm and upper arm. Look at your left palm (Figures 30-1, 30-2).

Notes: Your right heel touches the floor quickly. You should be exact when your fingers touch S12. Bend your legs slightly. Keep your torso upright. Relax your shoulders.

Effects: This prevents and treats nose disease, dizziness, headache, stomachache, sore throat and so on, and it also cleans the lungs and lets Qi (energy) through.

FORM 31 Scoop the Moon

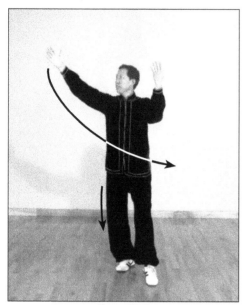

Figure 31-1

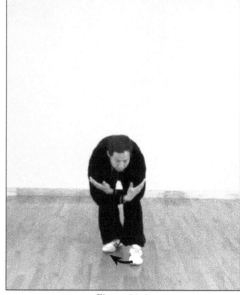

Figure 31-2

1. Keep both feet and left arm in the same position as above. Turn your torso to the right about ninety degrees, right hook forming a palm with fingers separated naturally. Then extend your right arm to the right side with your thumb pointing upward. Look at your right hand (Figure 31-1).

2. Bend your right knee as low as is comfortable. At the same time, turn your torso to the left about forty-five degrees, move your right hand downward, left, and up in a curve, crossing your forearms. Keep your right arm on the outside, right palm facing your forehead and left palm facing your right ear. Look at your right hand (Figure 31-2).

Notes: Your eyes follow your right hand as you move it. Your right hand follows your waist when you twist. All movements should be coordinated.

Effects: Prevents and relieves tennis elbow and pain in fingers, wrists, shoulders, waist, and back. Helps strengthen muscles in the legs.

FORM 32 Turn Body

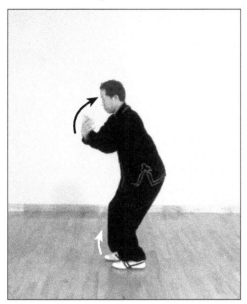 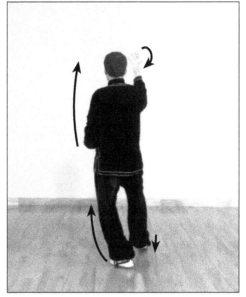

Figure 32-1   Figure 32-2

1. Turn your torso to the right about ninety degrees. Keep your right foot and both arms in the same position as above. Pivoting on your left heel, turn your left foot in until the big toes of both feet point at each other (Figure 32-1).

2. Shift your weight to your left foot as you turn right about sixty-five degrees. Pivoting on your right heel, turn your right foot outside to form a right empty stance. At the same time, raise your right arm slowly with your elbow bent until your palm faces your forehead. Point P8 of your right hand faces point GV24.5 of your head. Meanwhile, turn your left arm outside and pull inward until the small finger side touches CV17 point. Then press downward passing points CV15, CV13, CV10, S24, SP15, and G26 in order. Then turn your arm inside with your palm pressing the abdomen and down to the left side, palm facing upward. Look at your right palm (Figure 32-2).

Notes: Turning right should be coordinated with pressing your left hand down.

Effects: Prevents and relieves chest congestion, agitation, pain in waist and abdomen, and so on. It also regulates the balance of Yin and Yang.

FORM 33 Step Forward and Look at Wing

Shift your weight onto your right foot with your right knee bent. The left foot takes a step forward, touching the floor with the small toes. At the same time, turn your left arm outward until your palm faces forward and lift it upward with your elbow bent. Your left palm faces GV24.5. Meanwhile, extend your right arm slightly to the right until the palm faces your right temple. Look at your left hand (Figure 33-1).

Notes: Coordinate stepping with your left foot with raising your left arm.

Effects: Prevents and treats headache and eye diseases. It also clears away heat, expelling the "wind," refreshing the mind and brightening the eyes.

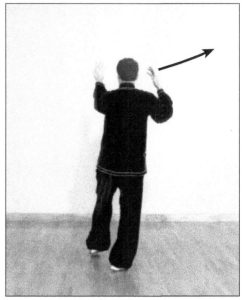

Figure 33-1

FORM 34 Look at the Moon

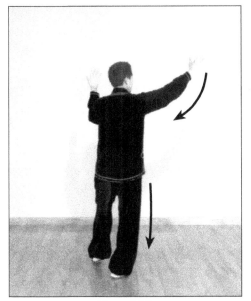

Figure 34-1

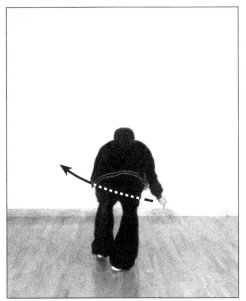

Figure 34-2

1. Both feet and left arm remain in the same position as above. Turn your torso to the right slightly and extend your right arm to the right side, thumb pointing upward. Look at your right hand (Figure 34-1).

2. Bend your right knee, controlling your balance. At the same time, turn your right arm inward until your palm faces down. Then bring it down and left in a curve to form a cross with your left arm. Your right palm faces point GV24.5. Your left palm faces your right temple. Then twist your torso to the left and look up at the sky (Figures 34-2, 34-3).

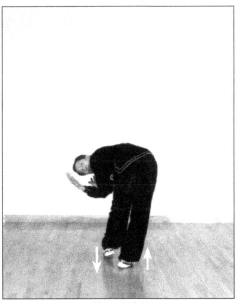

Figure 34-3

Notes: Keep your spine straight while you bend the torso forward and twist the waist to the left.

Effects: Prevents and treats dizziness, headache, ringing ears and pains in the neck, back, waist, and legs. It also relieves tiredness, dissipates the "wet" and cold, clears both the liver and gallbladder of obstruction, relaxes muscles and tendons, and makes joints pliable.

FORM 35 Press Air (Three Times)

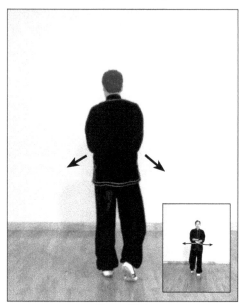

Figure 35-1

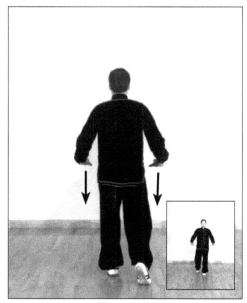

Figure 35-2

1. Raise your body and turn back to the center. Shift your weight onto the left foot with the entire sole on the floor. Raise your right heel off the floor. At the same time, both arms turn inward until your palms face downward. Cross your arms at the wrists and then press downward at each side of your knees. Keep your spine upright. Look straight ahead (Figures 35-1, 35-2).

2. Squat down until your hip sits on your right heel. Keep your spine erect as you lower your torso. At the same time, press your hands downward with palms facing down, thumbs and forefingers pointing toward each other. Keep your arms naturally bent. Look at your hands (Figure 35-3).

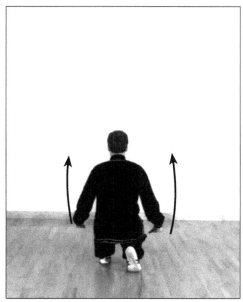

Figure 35-3

3. Then rise up until both legs are slightly bent. At the same time, bring your hands up level with the hips, keeping your elbows and wrists naturally relaxed, fingers a little bit lower than the wrists (see Figures 35-1, 35-2).

In this way, squat down and rise up two more times, a total of three times. Look at your hands (see Figures 35-2, 35-3, and 35-2 again).

Notes: Keep the same speed while squatting down and rising up. Breathe out when you squat down, breathe in when you rise up. Your weight rests mainly on the front foot.

Effect: It not only prevents and treats ringing in the ears, disorder in the intestines, stomach disorders, neck pain, back pain, waist pain, knee and ankle joint problems, but also strengthens the muscles of your legs.

FORM 36 Turn Body and Press Air (Three Times)

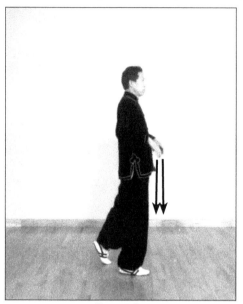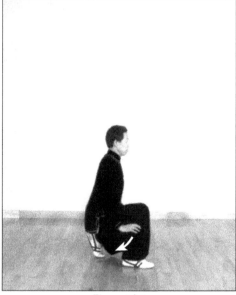

Figure 36-1	Figure 36-2

1. Keeping your arms in the same position (see Figure 35-2), turn ninety degrees to the right, pivoting on the balls of your feet. Shift your weight onto your right foot, keeping the entire sole on the floor. Raise your left heel off the floor. Look at your hands (Figure 36-1).

2. Squat down until your hip sits on your left heel. At the same time, both hands press down from both sides with palms facing down, thumbs and forefingers pointing at each other, fingers a bit higher than your wrists. Look at your hands (Figure 36-2).

In this way, rise up and squat down two more times (a total of three times).

Notes: Same as above, Form 35.

Effects: Same as above, Form 35.

FORM 37 Spread and Shake Wings

1. Rise up until your legs naturally straighten. Shift your weight onto your right foot with your left heel lifted off the floor. At the same time, with arms quivering, lift them forward to shoulder level, palms facing down, fingers pointing forward. Lean forward as far as you can. Look at your hands (Figures 37-1, 37-2).

2. Shift your weight onto your left foot, entire sole on the floor. Your right heel is lifted off the floor. At the same time, lift your arms upward until your palms face forward, fingers pointing upward with hands and arms quivering. Lean back as far as you can and look at your hands (Figures 37-3, 37-4).

Notes: Lifting your arms and shifting your weight should be coordinated. The range of quivering should be small; the frequency of quivering should be high.

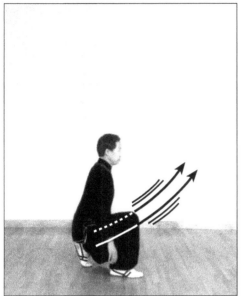

Figure 37-1

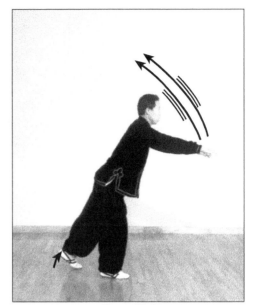

Figure 37-2

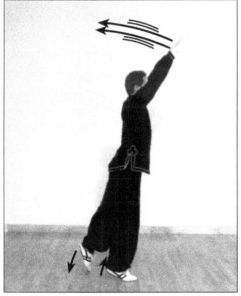

Figure 37-3

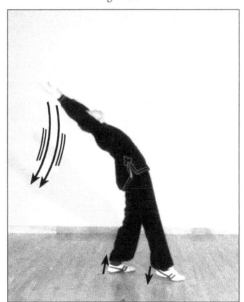

Figure 37-4

Effects: It can prevent and treat related diseases of the twelve channels, as well as promote good circulation to relax muscles and joints, clean fever and heal rheumatism, and strengthen intervillous or lesser circulation. It also has a good effect on terminal nerves and tiny blood vessels (capillaries).

FORM 38 Look Across at Water

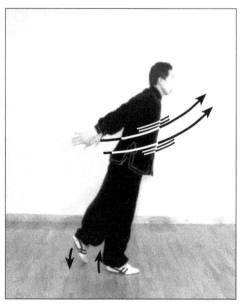 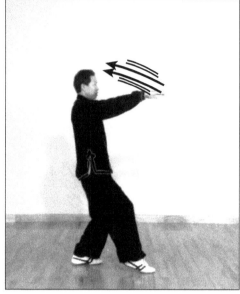

Figure 38-1   Figure 38-2

1. Shift your weight forward onto your right foot. Both knees are straightened and both heels are lifted off the floor. At the same time, both arms rotate inward while quivering them and lowering them from each side to the back in a curve, palms facing each other. Lean your body forward slightly. Look down to the front (Figure 38-1).

2. Then shift your weight on the left foot, with your knee bent and your foot flat on the floor. Your right heel is lifted off the floor. At the same time, quiver your arms while raising them forward and upward to shoulder level, palms facing down and fingers pointing forward. Look straight ahead (Figure 38-2).

Notes: Coordinate shifting your weight forward with lowering your arms behind you. Coordinate shifting your weight back with raising your arms forward to shoulder level.

Effects: This is good for cleaning fever and healing rheumatism.

FORM 39 Flying Bird Pats the Water (Left, Right, Left)

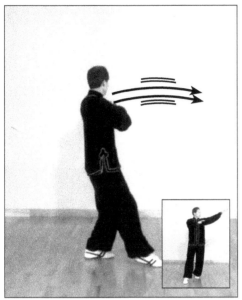

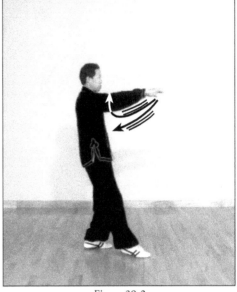

Figure 39-1   Figure 39-2

1. Pat Water Flying to Left Side:

Keep your weight on the left foot. Quiver both arms from the front to the left side, keeping your left hand at head level and the palm facing left. Keep your right hand at chest level with the palm facing downward. Look at your left hand (Figure 39-1).

2. Pat Water Flying to Right Side:

Turn to the right. Shift your weight onto your right foot, keeping it flat on the floor. Your left heel is lifted off the floor. Keep your knees straight. At the same time, quiver both arms while moving them from the left side to the right side. Your right hand is at head level with the palm facing right. Your left hand is at chest level with the palm facing downward. Both arms are bent slightly. Look at your right hand (Figures 39-2, 39-3).

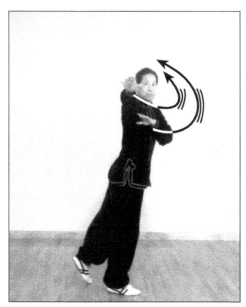

Figure 39-3

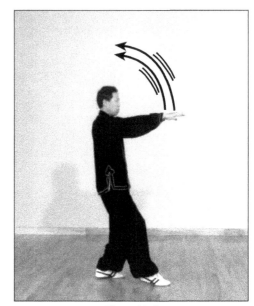

Figure 39-4

3. Pat Water Flying to Left Side:

(a.) Repeat #2 of this form, but reverse right and left (see Figure 39-1).

(b.) Turn your body back to the center, shifting your weight onto the right foot, entire sole on the floor. Lift your left heel off the floor, quivering both arms from the left side to center with palms facing downward at shoulder level. Look straight ahead (Figure 39-4).

Notes: All the movements must be continuous. Shifting your weight and quivering your arms must be coordinated.

Effects: This is good not only for cleaning fever and healing rheumatism, but it treats ringing ears and dizziness.

FORM 40 Drink Water (Three Times)

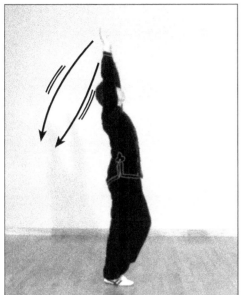
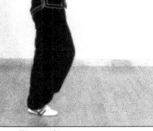
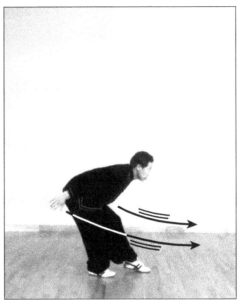

| Figure 40-1 | Figure 40-2 |

1. Shift your weight onto your right foot. Draw your left foot up to the right foot with the toes on the floor. At the same time, raise your quivering arms, palms facing forward. Look straight ahead (Figure 40-1).

2. Bend down on your right knee as far as is comfortable. Step forward with your left foot, the ball of the left foot on the floor. At the same time, bring both hands down from both sides, palms facing each other (Figure 40-2).

Then reach both hands down and forward from both sides of the left leg to the front of the left foot with quivering arms, palms facing downward, fingers pointing forward. Bend at the waist and lean your torso forward while keeping your head lifted up and looking down to the front (Figure 40-3).

3. Continuing the last movement, raise your torso upright. Lift both arms upward and backward to shoulder level, then separate the quivering arms to the sides with palms facing downward. Bring both hands to each side of your hips, palms facing each other. Look straight ahead (Figures 40-4, 40-5, 40-6).

4. Lean your torso forward, reaching both hands down and forward from both sides of your left leg to the front of your left foot with quivering arms, palms facing downward, fingers pointing forward, head lifted up and looking down to the front (see Figure 40-3).

5. Repeat steps #3 and #4 of this form one more time (a total of three times).

Notes: The movements must be continuous, natural, coordinated, and steady.

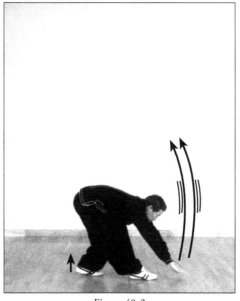

Figure 40-3

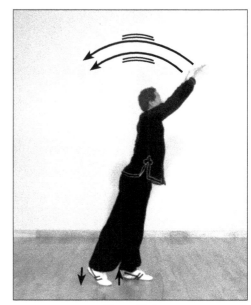

Figure 40-4

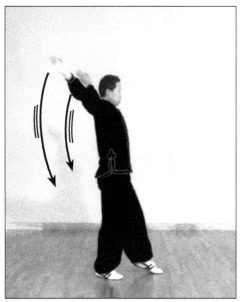
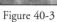

Figure 40-5

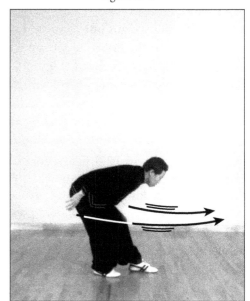

Figure 40-6

Effects: Strengthens the legs, dredges the three Yang and Yin Channels of the foot, and helps remove disease from the feet.

FORM 41 Look at the Sky

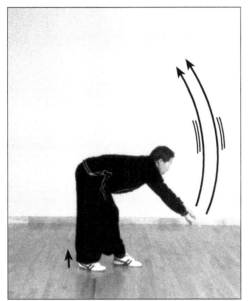

Figure 41-1

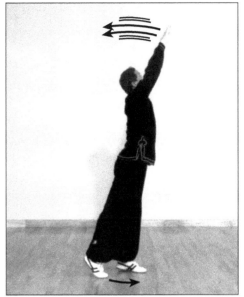

Figure 41-2

Shift your weight onto your left foot and straighten your left leg. Keep your left foot flat on the floor. Your right heel is lifted off the floor. At the same time, lift your hands upward, raising your torso slowly and quivering your arms quickly, palms facing forward, thumbs pointing toward each other. Look at the sky (Figures 41-1, 41-2).

Notes: Shifting your weight and quivering your arms must be coordinated with slowly raising your torso.

Effects: Relaxes the muscles and joints, clears the channels and joints, and helps get rid of diseases.

FORM 42 Recover Qi

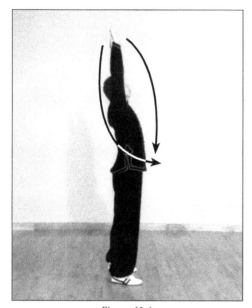

Figure 42-1

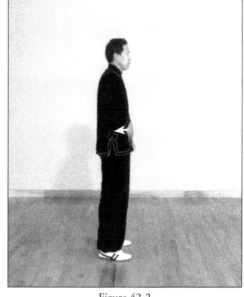

Figure 42-2

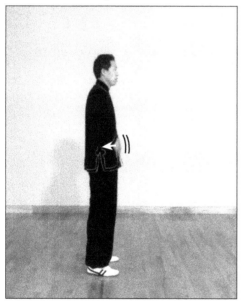

Figure 42-3

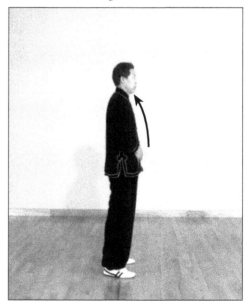

Figure 42-4

Move your right foot to a position parallel with your left foot, keeping both feet shoulder-width apart. Your weight is distributed equally on both legs. At the same time, bring both arms upward, still quivering, down to both sides of the Dantian. Place your left hand to the lower left of the Dantian with the fingers apart. Place your

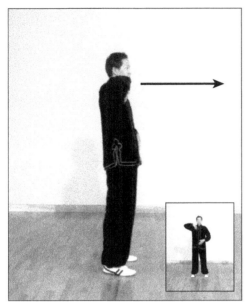

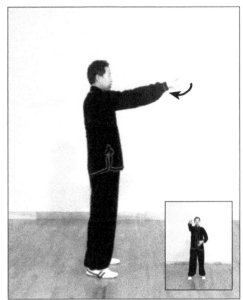

Figure 43-1   Figure 43-2

right hand to the lower right of the Dantian with the fingers apart. The thumbs of each hand point toward each other (Figures 42-1, 42-2). Then shake your stomach three times, pausing a few seconds between each shake. Look straight ahead (Figures 42-3, 42-4).

Notes: Stepping with your right foot and bending your arms down to both sides of the Dantian must be coordinated. Relax your shoulders and elbows when you shake your stomach with your hands.

Effects: Helps clear the Qi of the stomach, liver, and spleen. Helps to remove the diseases from the body.

FORM 43 Grasp Air (Ten Times)

1. Without moving your feet, raise your right hand to your S13 point (Figure 43-1). Then, reach out with your right hand to the front at shoulder level, twisting your right shoulder forward, palm facing down. Look straight ahead (Figure 43-2).

2. Curl the fingers of your right hand in to form a "hollow fist," leaving a hollow space between your fingers and palm. Look ahead (Figure 43-3).

3. Draw your right fist backward to within one inch from your chest just under

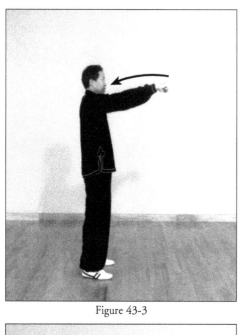

Figure 43-3

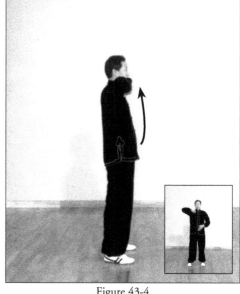

Figure 43-4

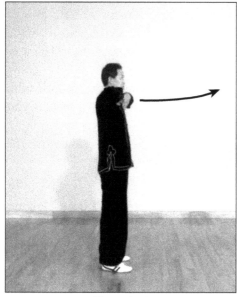

Figure 43-5

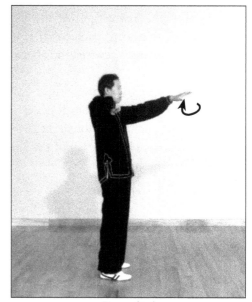
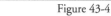

Figure 43-6

the collar bone, with the thumb side of the hollow fist (Quan Yan) facing the right S13 (Qihu) point. Relax your right shoulder and keep your armpit empty, elbow pointing outside. At the same time, raise your left hand to your left S13 point (Figures 43-4, 43-5). Then, reach out with your left hand to the front at shoulder level, twisting your left shoulder forward, palm facing down. Look ahead (Figure 43-6).

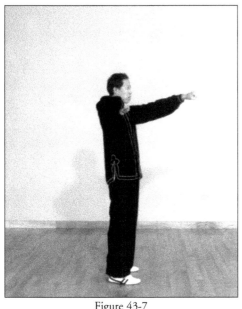

Figure 43-7

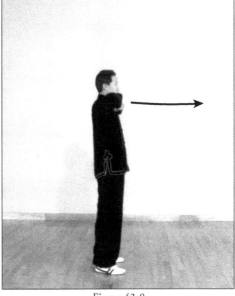

Figure 43-8

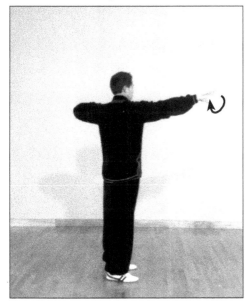

Figure 43-9

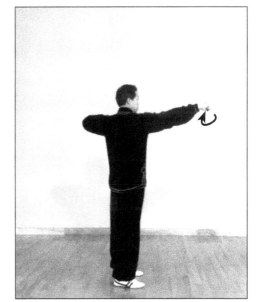

Figure 43-10

4. Repeat #2 of this form with the left hand (Figures 43-7 through 43-14).

5. Repeat eight times more, alternating right and left. Do the Grasp Air movement a total of ten times.

Notes: Relax your shoulders and keep your armpits empty when you do the Grasp Air movements. Keep your spine straight when you twist your waist.

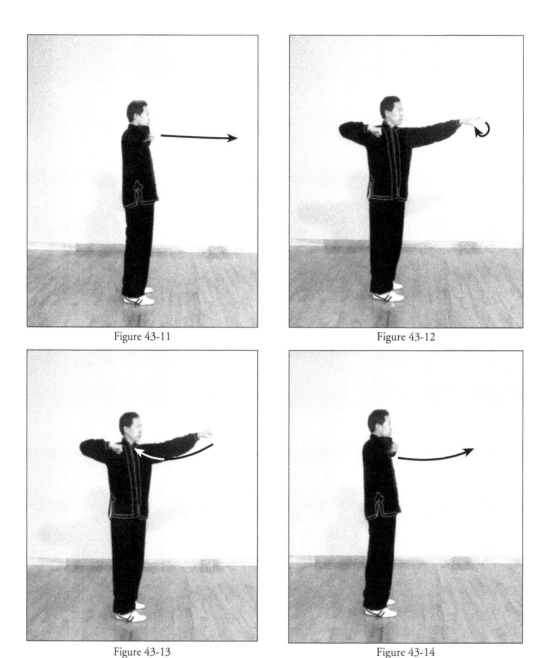

Figure 43-11

Figure 43-12

Figure 43-13

Figure 43-14

Effects: Receive energy from nature. This helps relieve fever, clears the channels, stops pain, extends the chest and lets the energy circulate, and also treats some diseases such as cough, asthma, chest pain, back pains, waist pain, and so on.

FORM 44 Grasp Air With Palm Up (Ten Times)

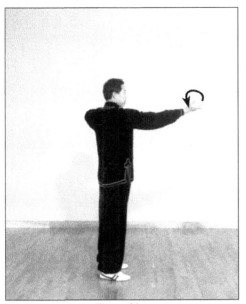

Figure 44-1

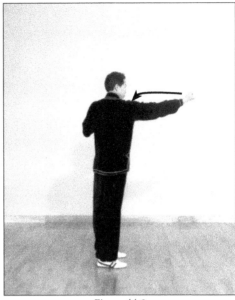

Figure 44-2

1. Keep your feet in the same position as above. Turn your right arm outward and stretch it forward, straightening your arm and your palm facing upward. Look ahead (Figure 44-1).

2. Curl the fingers of your right hand to form a "hollow fist," leaving a hollow space between your fingers and palm. Look ahead (Figure 44-2).

3. Draw your right fist backward to within one inch from your chest just under your collar bone, little finger side of your hollow fist facing the right S13 (Qihu) point. Relax your shoulder with your right elbow pointed downward. Your right palm faces the right side (Figure 44-3). At the same time, turn your left arm outward and stretch it forward, straightening your arm and your palm facing upward. Look ahead (Figure 44-4).

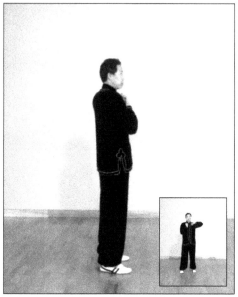

Figure 44-3

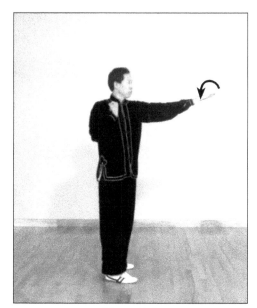

Figure 44-4

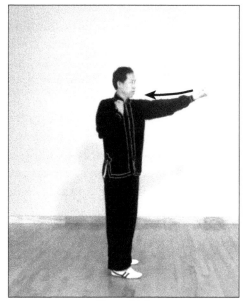

Figure 44-5

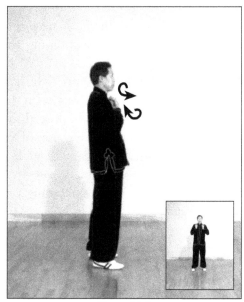

Figure 44-6

4. Repeat #2 of this form with your right hand (Figure 44-5).

5. Repeat eight times more, alternating right and left. Do the Grasp Air with Palm Up movements a total of ten times (Figure 44-6).

Notes: Relax your shoulders and point your elbows down. Twist your waist and hips.

Effects: Same as Form 43, Grasp Air.

FORM 45 Holding a Ball

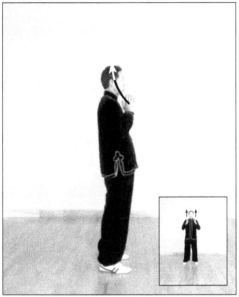

Figure 45-1

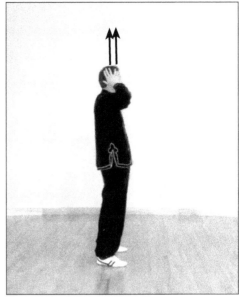

Figure 45-2

1. Keep the position of your feet the same as above. Bend your elbows and turn your arms inward until your palms face each other. Thumbs point toward your chest (Figure 45-1).

2. With both palms facing your ears, thrust your fingers upward. Keep your arms straight and palms facing each other. Relax your shoulders. Look at your hands (Figures 45-2, 45-3).

3. Turn your arms outward until your palms face outside, and then bring them down from both sides in a curve to the front of your feet. As you bring your arms down, bend your torso forward about ninety degrees. The fingers of each hand point at each other, palms facing upward, as if holding a ball. Keep your legs straight. The GV20 (Baihui) point faces forward. Look at your hands (Figures 45-4, 45-5, 45-6).

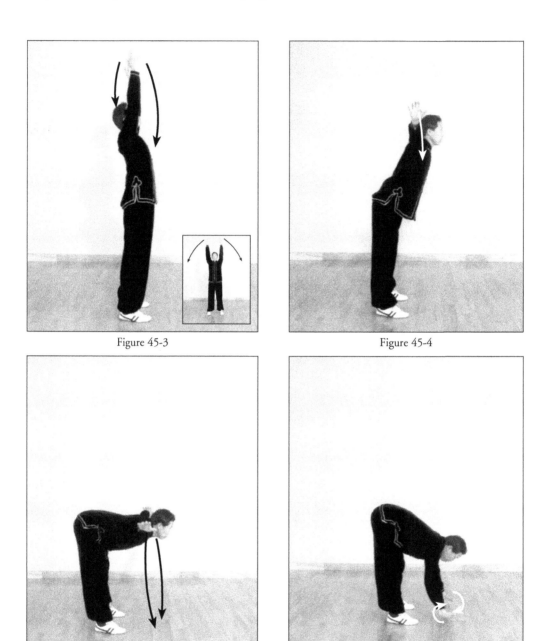

Figure 45-3

Figure 45-4

Figure 45-5

Figure 45-6

Notes: Keep your spine and legs straight, slightly bending your elbows and wrists as if holding a big ball.

Effects: Receive energy from nature. Speeds up blood circulation.

FORM 46 Rotate (Knead) the Ball

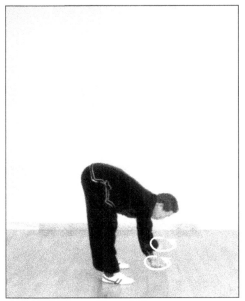

Figure 46-1

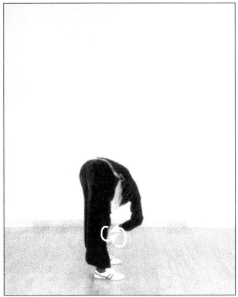

Figure 46-2

1. Keep your feet in the same position. Raise your torso slightly. At the
same time, both hands hold a ball in
front of you as low as you can. Then
turn your right arm inward, bending your elbow, until your palm faces
down. Turn your left arm outward
until your palm faces up. Palms face
each other about eight inches apart, as
if you are holding an imaginary ball.
Look at your hands (Figure 46-1).

2. Turn your torso to the left about
ninety degrees. At the same time, imagine yourself rotating the ball at a level
and counter-clockwise direction. Rotate
the ball about two circles to your left
side. Look at your hands (Figure 46-2).

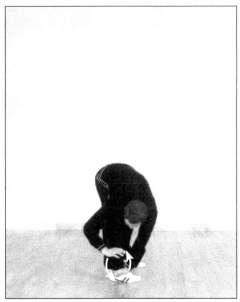

Figure 46-3

3. As you turn your torso to the
right about 180 degrees, continue rotating the ball at the same level and in a counter-
clockwise direction. Rotate the ball about eight circles to your right side. Look at
your hands (Figure 46-3).

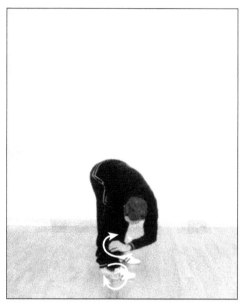

Figure 47-1

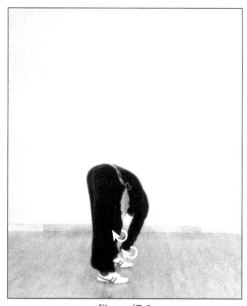

Figure 47-2

Notes: Let your waist lead your shoulders, shoulders lead elbows, elbows lead wrists, and wrists lead fingers when you are rotating the ball. The whole movement must be coordinated and combined.

Effects: Clears the channels and joints of your hands. Supplies energy to benefit the kidneys and Yuan-qi, helps blood circulation, adjusts effects of viscera, and increases the flexibility of the joints of the arms, legs, and waist.

FORM 47 Turn Body and Rotate Ball

1. Keep the position of your feet the same as above. Turn both arms until your left hand is on the top, right hand under your left hand, palms facing each other, eight inches apart. Look at your hands (Figure 47-1).

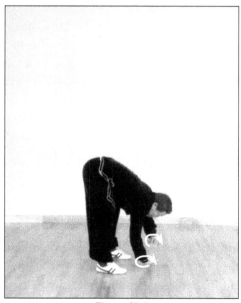

Figure 47-3

2. Then turn your torso to left about 180 degrees. At the same time, imagine yourself rotating the ball in a clockwise direction and keeping it at the same level. Rotate the ball about eight revolutions to your left side. Look at your hands (Figure 47-2).

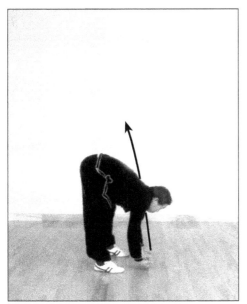

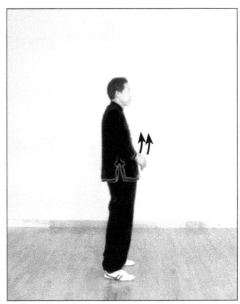

| Figure 47-4 | Figure 47-5 |

3. Then turn your torso to the right about ninety degrees. While continuously rotating the ball at a level and in a clockwise direction, rotate the ball about two revolutions to the center. Look at your hands (Figure 47-3).

4. Raise your torso, turn both arms in, bending your elbows, until your palms face your abdomen. Look straight ahead (Figures 47-4, 47-5).

Notes: Same as Form 46.

Effects: Same as Form 46.

FORM 48 Holding Air

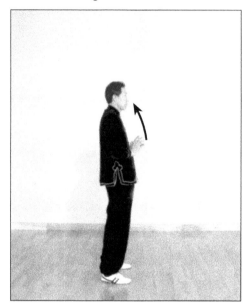

Figure 48-1

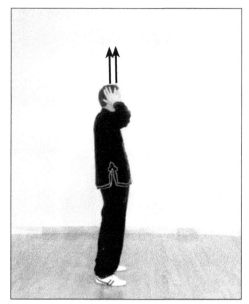

Figure 48-2

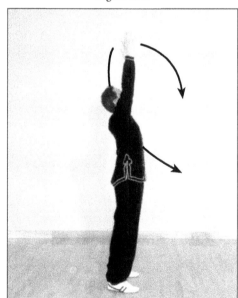

Figure 48-3

1. Keep the position of your feet the same as above. Lift your arms up until they are straight, palms facing each other, fingers pointing up. Look at your hands (Figures 48-1, 48-2, 48-3).

2. Turn both arms outward until your left palm faces left, right palm faces right. Then bring your hands down to both sides in a curve with your knees straightened naturally. At the same time, bend your torso forward about ninety degrees, with G20 (Baihui) point facing forward (Figure 48-4).

Then flex your wrists as you lower your hands in front of your feet. Your fingers point at each other and palms face upward, as though holding a bulky weight. Look forward and down (Figure 48-5).

3. Squat down as low as you can, keeping both feet flat on the floor. At the same time, lift your torso upward until your spine is straight. Lift your arms up to shoulder level with the fingers of each hand pointing at each other and palms facing your chest. Look ahead (Figure 48-6).

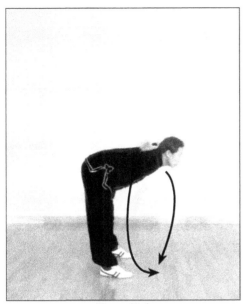

Figure 48-4

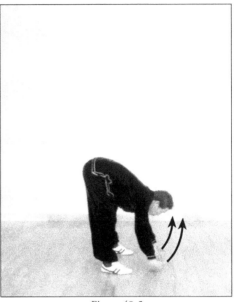

Figure 48-5

Notes: Bend forward as far as you feel comfortable, but do not bend your knees until you bring your hands from both sides down in front of your feet. Move slowly when you stand up.

Effects: Speeds blood circulation and improves the power and flexibility of the legs.

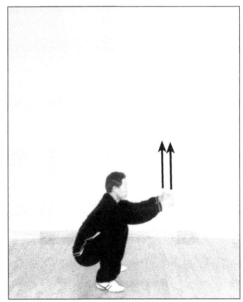

Figure 48-6

FORM 49 Go Through Air

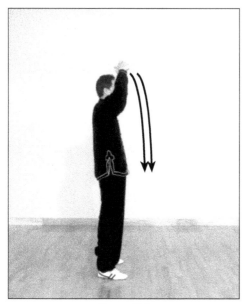

Figure 49-1

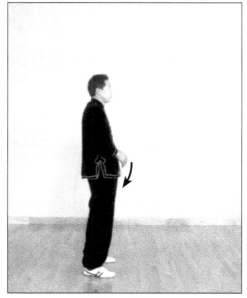

Figure 49-2

1. Keep the position of your feet the same as above. Keep your arms in the same position as you stand up. Look ahead.

Raise your hands upward and inward until your palms are facing your temples, fingers pointing at each other, four inches apart. Look ahead (Figure 49-1).

2. Slowly lower your hands down past your chest to your lower Dantian for a few seconds. Look ahead (Figure 49-2).

3. Then slowly lower your hands and let your arms hang down at both sides. Look straight ahead (Figure 49-3).

Notes: Let your mind lead your movements. Keep your whole body naturally relaxed.

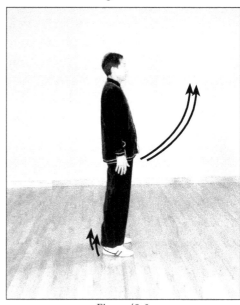

Figure 49-3

Effects: Provides energy to the body from upper, middle and lower Dantian in order to benefit Tiyin. It also clears the mind, brightens the eyes, warms the body and makes you feel comfortable.

FORM 50 Raise Wings

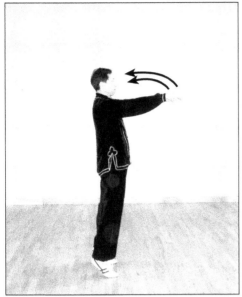

Figure 50-1

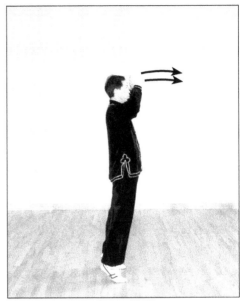

Figure 50-2

1. Lift both heels off the floor slowly. At the same time, raise both hands forward and upward to shoulder level, palms facing down (Figure 50-1).

Then raise your hands upward and turn your arms inward, bending your elbows, until your hands are in front of your forehead. Your thumbs point at each other, palms face forward, and your elbows are bent about ninety degrees and point out to each side. Look at your hands (Figure 50-2).

2. Both heels touch the floor quickly when your hands push forward and upward with your wrists flexed back, thumbs pointing at each other. Look at your hands (Figure 50-3).

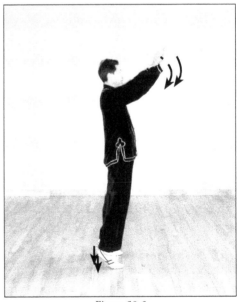

Figure 50-3

Notes: Coordinate lifting your heels and raising your hands. Your heels touch the floor simultaneously with pushing your hands forward. The whole movement should be continuous and harmonious, relaxing your shoulders and sinking your elbows.

Effects: Keeps the balance of Yin and Yang.

FORM 51 Drop Wings

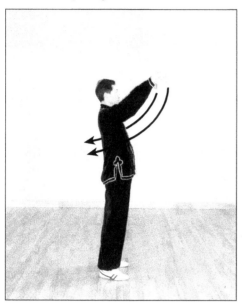

Figure 51-1

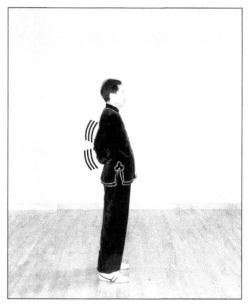

Figure 52-1

Keep the position of your feet and arms the same as above. Wrists bend forward and down, the tips of your fingers together, fingers pointing downward. Look ahead (Figure 51-1).

Notes: Your whole body must be relaxed naturally; particularly, sink your shoulders.

Effects: Removes stagnant Qi from the tips of the fingers and also draws more energy from both G30 (Huantiao) points.

FORM 52 Place Wings on the Back

Keep the position of your feet the same as above. Both hands extend to the sides, downward and backward in a curve with elbows bent about ninety degrees so that both LI4 (Hegu) points

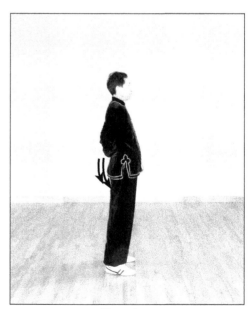

Figure 52-2

of your hands are placed on the B23 (shenyu) points. Your palms are facing up with the fingers separated naturally. Then shake your hands seven times. Pause a few seconds, then shake seven times again. Repeat this pause and shaking sequence seven times once more. Look straight ahead (Figures 52-1, 52-2).

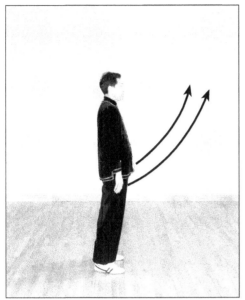

Figure 53-1

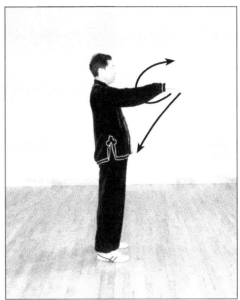

Figure 53-2

Notes: Keep Baihua point straight upward (perpendicular), neck erect, and shoulders relaxed. Let your elbows hang and relax your waist.

Effects: Benefits the kidneys, strengthens energies, clears away heat, and disperses wetness. It also treats diseases of the reproductive system, kidney disease, waist and back pain, emission, impotence, and so on.

FORM 53 Fly Up from Side to Side (Seven Times)

1. Keep the position of your feet the same as above. Bring both hands down past G30 (Huantiao) points by your sides (Figure 53-1), letting your arms hang down naturally. Look straight ahead.

2. Then raise your hands in front of you up to shoulder level, palms facing down, fingers pointing forward and spread apart naturally. Look ahead (see Figure 53-2).

3. Fly up to left: Turn your torso slightly to the left, shift your weight to the right foot with your knee bent. Step with your left foot, the small toe touching the floor first. At the same time, your right hand presses down in a curve and stops about one inch in front of the lower Dantian, palm facing inward. Raise your left hand to the left, with your elbow slightly bent, to head level. Your palm faces the Yiantang point. Your thumb points up and the other four fingers point right. Your fingers are spread apart naturally. Look at your left hand (Figure 53-3).

4. Fly up to right: Turn your torso slightly to the right, shifting your weight to the left foot with your knee bent and bring your right foot next to your left (Figure 53-4). Step forward with your right foot, the small toe touching the floor first. At the

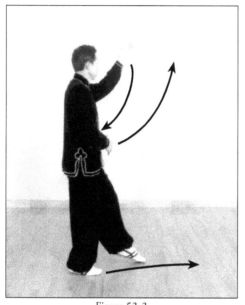

Figure 53-3

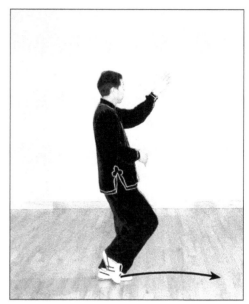

Figure 53-4

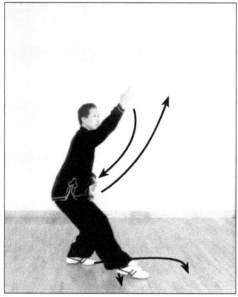

Figure 53-5

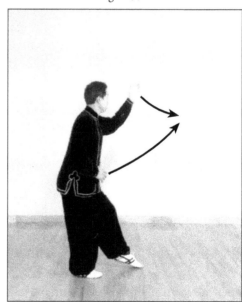

Figure 53-6

same time, your left hand presses down in a curve and stops about one inch in front of the lower Dantian, palm facing inward. Raise your right hand forty-five degrees between center and right with your elbow slightly bent to head level. Your palm faces the Yiantaing point. Your thumb points up and the other four fingers point left. Your fingers are spread apart naturally. Look at your right hand (Figure 53-5).

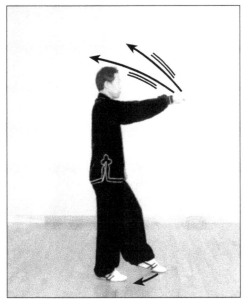
Figure 54-1

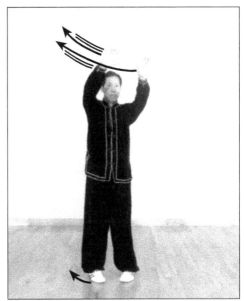
Figure 54-2

In this way, do Fly Up movement a total of seven times, alternating left and right steps. The last movement is the same as Fly Up to left of this form (Figure 53-6).

Notes: Stepping must be coordinated with hand movements. When your left foot steps forward, raise your left hand, and when your right foot steps forward, raise your right hand.

Effects: It not only benefits energy, adjusts the nerves of the vertebrae, cleans fever and relieves rheumatism, but also strengthens legs and improves coordination of limbs and body.

FORM 54 Turn Body

1. Keep the position of your feet the same as above. Turn your torso back to the center. Drop your left arm down to chest level. Raise your right arm forward and upward to chest level, keeping your arms straight naturally and shoulder-width apart. Relax your shoulders and wrists, palms facing down, fingers pointing forward. Look straight ahead (Figure 54-1).

2. Turn right about ninety degrees, keeping your legs bent. Turn your left foot inward about 135 degrees so you are standing "pigeon toed," keeping your left heel on the floor. Distribute your weight equally on both legs. At the same time, raise your arms up to head level and quiver your arms (Figure 54-2).

Notes: Coordinate turning your left toes inward, turning your torso and swinging your arms to the right about ninety degrees.

Effects: Improves coordination of your arms and legs.

FORM 55 Fanning Upward

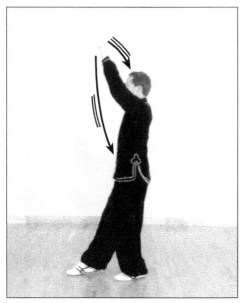
Figure 55-1

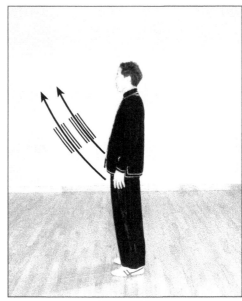
Figure 55-2

1. Shift your weight on your left foot as you turn right ninety degrees. Your right foot turns out about 135 degrees, keeping your right heel on the floor. Then lift your right heel off the floor. At the same time, raise your arms up to the right until they straighten and continue shaking them. Your palms face forward and your fingers point up. Look straight ahead (Figure 55-1).

2. Keep the position of your feet the same as above. Shake your arms as you drop them down by your sides. Let your arms hang naturally. Look ahead (Figure 55-2).

Notes: Coordinate turning your right foot outward with raising your arms.

Effects: It prevents and treats waist and back pain, pain in the ribs, bloated stomach, and congested chest.

FORM 56 Fly Over the Water (Seven Times)

1. Keep your feet the same as above while quivering your arms, raise them forward to shoulder level. Look straight ahead (Figure 56-1).

2. Fly Over the Water to the Left:

Turn your torso to the left about forty-five degrees, bending your right knee. Step forward with your left foot with the small toe of your left foot touching the floor and your knee bent slightly. At the same time, bring your quivering arms in a curve to the left. Your left arm goes to the upper left and comes above head level with the palm facing left and thumb pointing down. Your right hand goes to the left side at chest level with the palm facing down and fingers pointing left. Both arms are bent naturally. Look at your left hand (Figure 56-2).

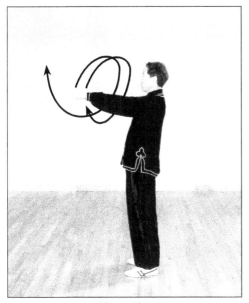

Figure 56-1

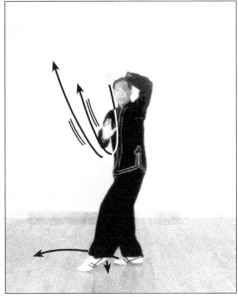

Figure 56-2

3. Fly Over Water to the Right:

Turn your torso to the right about forty-five degrees. Shift your weight forward onto the left foot with your knee bent. The right foot steps forward with the small toe of this foot touching the floor and your knee bent slightly. At the same time, bring your quivering arms in a curve to the right. Your right arm goes to the upper right and comes above head level with the palm facing right, thumb pointing downward; your left hand goes to the right side at chest level, with the palm facing down and fingers pointing right. Both arms are bent naturally. Look at your right hand (Figure 56-3).

4. In this way, do Fly Over the Water movement a total of seven times. The last movement of this form is the same as Fly Over the Water to the Left (Figure 56-4).

Notes: Bring your arms in a curve to the right when you take a step to the right, bring your arms in a curve to the left when you take a step to the left. Your arms must be coordinated with your footwork.

Effects: It relaxes muscles and makes joints pliable, strengthens the muscles of your legs, and benefits the waist and lower back.

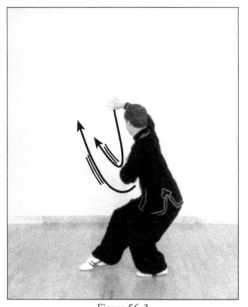

Figure 56-3

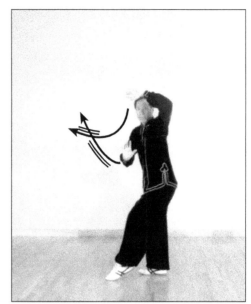

Figure 56-4

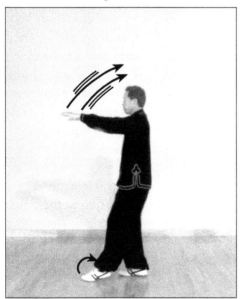

Figure 57-1

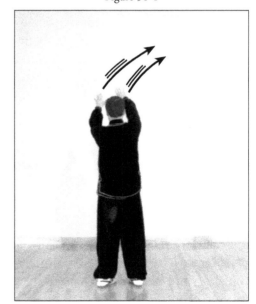

Figure 57-2

FORM 57 Turn Body

Repeat Form 54, Turn Body, but reverse right and left (Figures 57-1, 57-2).

Notes: Same as Form 54.

Effects: Same as Form 54.

FORM 58 Fly Up

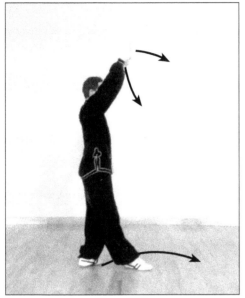

Figure 58-1

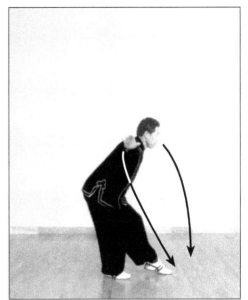

Figure 59-1

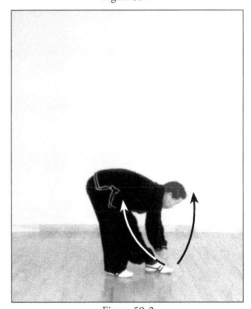

Figure 59-2

Repeat Form 55, Fanning Upward, but reverse right and left (Figure 58-1).

Notes: Same as Form 55.

Effects: Same as Form 55.

FORM 59 Look for Food (Seven Times)

1. Look for Food to the Left Side:

(a.) Bend your right knee as low as possible and step forward with your left foot, the ball of the foot touching the floor first; your left knee is bent naturally and your torso bends forward. At the same time, bring your arms from both sides to the front, and then cross them in front of your left knee or foot. The left arm is on top, your left hand points to the right, and your right hand points to the left. Both palms face downward (Figures 59-1, 59-2).

(b.) Keep the position of your feet the same as above. Raise your torso slightly. At the same time, swing both arms back to each side with your arms turned outside,

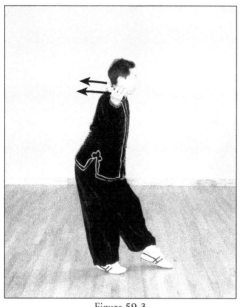

Figure 59-3

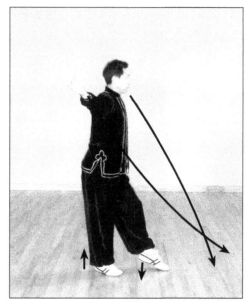

Figure 59-4

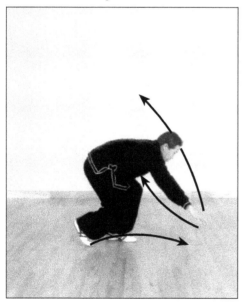

Figure 59-5

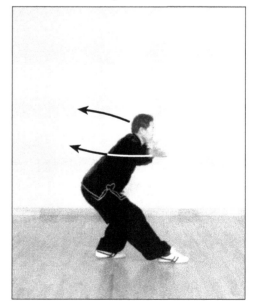

Figure 59-6

palms facing upward, thumbs pointing backward. Keep your hands at shoulder level. Look straight ahead (Figures 59-3, 59-4).

2. Look for Food to the Right Side:

Repeat #1 above, reversing left and right (Figures 59-5, 59-6, 59-7).

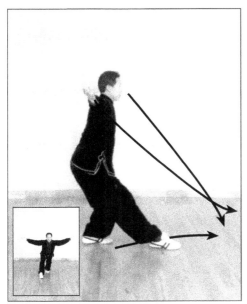

Figure 59-7

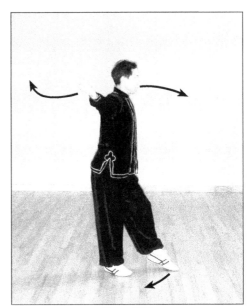

Figure 59-8

3. In this way, do Look for Food a total of seven times, ending with Look for Food to the Left Side (see Figure 59-8).

Notes: Keep your spine straight when your torso is leaning forward. At the same time, extend your arms as far as possible. Bend your knee as low as you feel comfortable.

Effects: Helps prevent and treat waist pain, back pain, spine pain, fever, cough, and asthma; strengthens legs, improves the coordination and flexibility of limbs, and makes them pliable and strong.

FORM 60 Turn Body

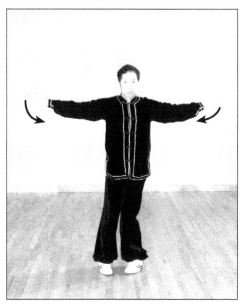

Figure 60-1

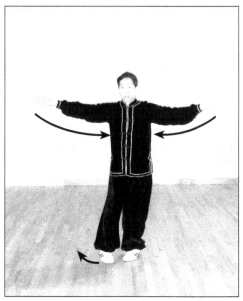

Figure 60-2

1. Turn your torso to the right about ninety degrees. Turn your left foot inward about 135 degrees with the heel as the axis. Shift your weight so it is evenly distributed on both legs. At the same time, turn both arms inward, palms facing down. Look straight ahead (Figures 60-1, 60-2).

2. Shift your weight onto your left leg. Turn your right foot out about 135 degrees with the heel as the axis. Then the ball of your right foot touches on the floor with the right heel lifted off the floor. At the same time, bend both arms by your left side with palms facing down and at chest level. Fingers are pointing at each other. Look at your hands (Figure 60-3).

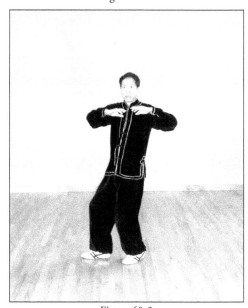

Figure 60-3

Notes: Coordinate turning your left foot inward with turning both arms inward. Coordinate turning your right foot outward with bending both arms.

Effects: Turn body, in order to train Dai-channel as you receive the great energy from the Laogong point and sink the Qi in the lower Dantian.

FORM 61 Look for the Nest (Left, Middle, Right, Right, Middle, Left, and Left)

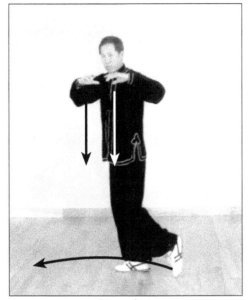 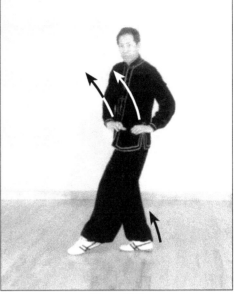

Figure 61-1   Figure 61-2

1. Left Style

Shift your weight onto your right foot with your knee bent. Your left foot steps forward with the ball of your foot touching the floor first. At the same time, press your palms down to the side of your left hip. The forefinger and thumb of each hand are pointing toward each other about one inch apart. Your palms face down. Look at your hands (Figures 61-1, 61-2).

2. Middle Style

Shift your weight onto your left foot with your knee bent and bring your right heel off the floor with the toes on the floor. At the same time, turn your torso back to the center. Lift both hands in front of the chest with elbows bent. Relax the wrists and shoulders (Figure 61-3).

Then your right foot steps forward with the ball of the foot touching the floor first. At the same time, press both palms down in front of your abdomen, palms facing down, fingers of each hand pointing toward each other. Look at your hands (Figure 61-4).

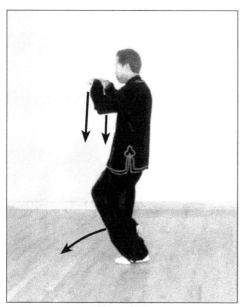

Figure 61-3

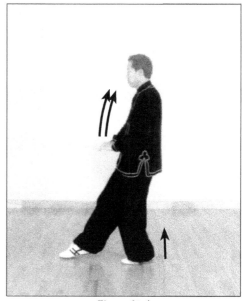

Figure 61-4

3. Right Style

Shift your weight onto your right foot with your right knee bent, and bring your left heel off the floor with the toes on the floor. At the same time, turn your torso to the right. Raise both hands up to chest level with your elbows bent and wrists relaxed (Figure 61-5).

Then your left foot steps forward with the ball of the foot touching the floor first. At the same time, press both palms down to the side of your right hip, palms facing down and fingers of each hand pointing toward each other. Look at your hands (Figure 61-6).

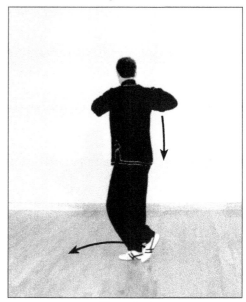

Figure 61-5

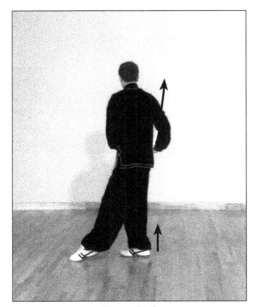

Figure 61-6

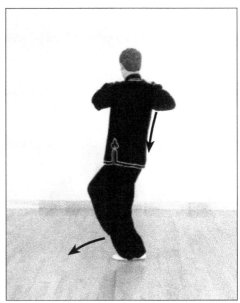

Figure 61-7

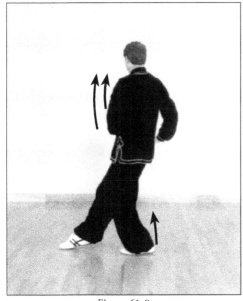

Figure 61-8

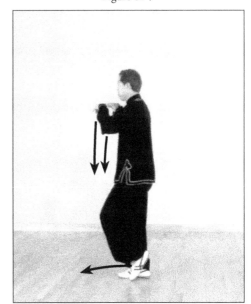

Figure 61-9

4. Right Style

Repeat #3 of this form, but step forward with your right foot (Figures 61-7, 61-8).

5. Middle Style

Repeat #2 of this form, but step forward with your left foot (Figures 61-9, 61-10).

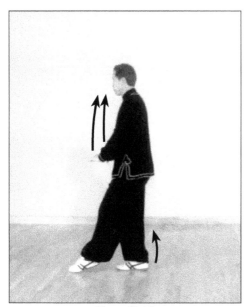

Figure 61-10

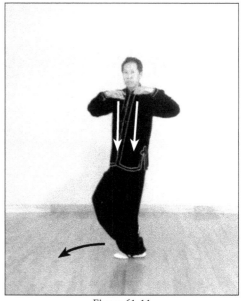

Figure 61-11

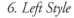

6. Left Style

Repeat #1 of this form, but step forward with your right foot (Figures 61-11, 61-12).

7. Left Style

Repeat #1 of this form. (see Figure 61-1).

Notes: Coordinate shifting your weight with raising your hands. Coordinate stepping forward with pressing your palms down. Do not raise your hands higher than the middle Dantian. Press your palms down no lower than your hips.

Effects: The middle Dantian receives the energy from nature. This form helps to remove the diseases from the palms, fingers, and wrists.

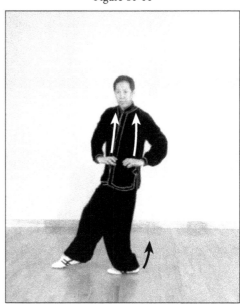

Figure 61-12

FORM 62 Turn Body and Shake (Quiver) Wings

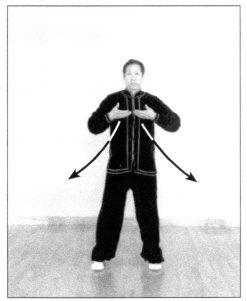

Figure 62-1

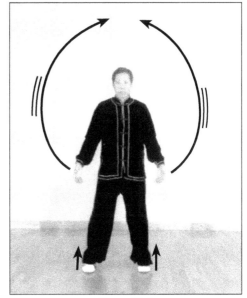

Figure 62-2

1. Take a step forward with your right foot. At the same time, turn your body to the left ninety degrees, using the balls of your feet as the axis. Keeping your feet flat on the floor, shift your weight between your legs. Keep your feet parallel and shoulder-width apart. At the same time, turn your palms outward until they face upward. Look ahead (Figure 62-1).

2. Lower your hands to your sides (Figure 62-2). Lift both heels slightly off the floor as you raise both hands from your sides over your head with your arms quivering. Your palms are facing each other. Look at your hands (Figure 62-3).

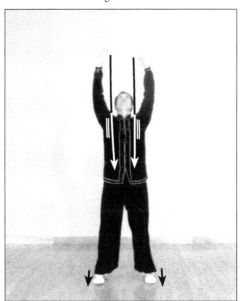

Figure 62-3

3. Heels touch on the floor when you press both palms down in front of your abdomen with arms quivering, palms facing your abdomen, and fingers of both hands pointing at each other. Then your arms stop quivering. Look straight ahead (Figure 62-4).

Notes: Your arms lead your hands, naturally quivering. Relax your waist and shoulders when you raise your arms.

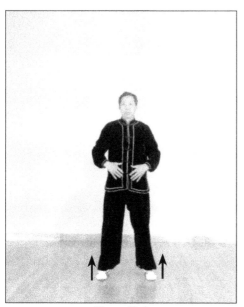

Figure 62-4

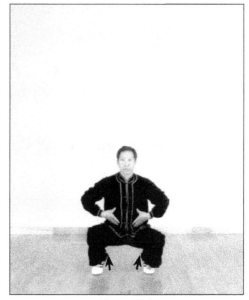

Figure 63-1

Effects: Receive nature's energy from upper Dantian, middle Dantian, and lower Dantian.

FORM 63 Sleep Peacefully and Recover Air

1. Squat down with your heels off the floor. Both thumbs press S18 points at each side. The other four fingers of each hand press each side of the lower Dantian, keeping one inch between your hands. Look straight ahead (Figure 63-1).

2. Keeping your feet and hands in the same position as above, bend your torso slightly forward and lower your head in meditation for about thirty seconds. Look forward and down about three feet in front of you (Figure 63-2).

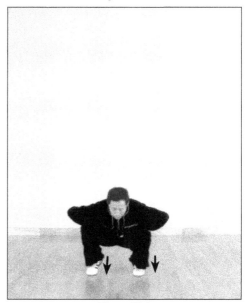

Figure 63-2

Notes: Relax your entire body. Your torso does not lean forward too much. Concentrate on the lower Dantian. Squat down as low as feels comfortable to you.

Effects: Receive nature's energy from upper Dantian. Gathers internal energy at the lower Dantian so that energy is recovered.

FORM 64 Closing Posture

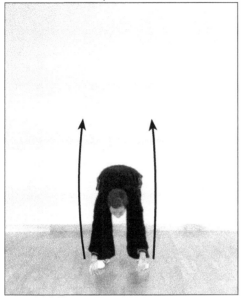

Figure 64-1

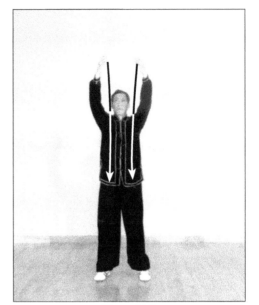

Figure 64-2

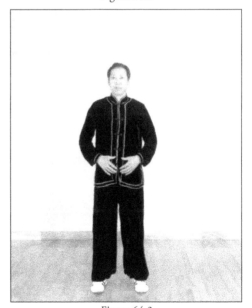

Figure 64-3

1. Raise your hips up slowly, straightening your knees and with your heels on the floor. Lean your torso forward with your spine straight. At the same time, both arms straighten, with palms facing forward. Look forward and down (Figure 64-1).

2. Your legs keep the same position as above. Raise your torso up slowly until your spine is erect. At the same time, raise both arms slowly forward and up, palms facing each other and fingers pointing up. Look at your hands (Figure 64-2).

3. Turn both palms inside, fingers of each hand pointing at each other. Then bring your hands slowly down past your temples, chest, and abdomen to the sides. Relax your shoulders, arms, and hands. Sink the internal Qi to the Dantian. Look ahead (Figure 64-3).

4. Bring your left foot next to your right foot and stand at attention. Look straight ahead (Figures 64-4, 64-5).

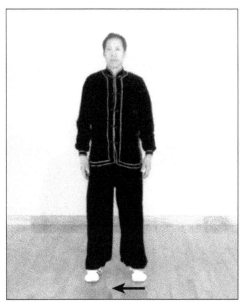
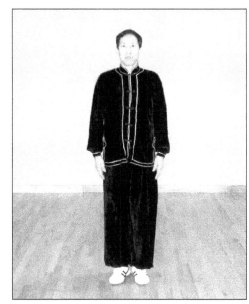

| Figure 64-4 | Figure 64-5 |

Notes: Lean your torso forward only as low as you feel comfortable. Raise your hips or torso slowly so that you don't become dizzy. Keep your arms and spine naturally straight.

Effects: Receive energy from nature so that it benefits the Yuanqi of lower Dantian.

Conclusion

Persevere in Wild Goose Qigong exercise. This not only improves mental and physical strength, but also can heal diseases. If diseases are absent, it may prevent their developing. It also helps you recover from fatigue, maintain physical fitness, delay aging, and prolong life.

References

1. *The Chinese Wushu Dictionary,* p. 9, (1990) Chinese Sports Publishing House.

2. Ibid.

3. Ibid.

4. Jiren Ma, *Chinese Qigong*, (1983) Shanxi Science and Technology Publishing House.

5. Ibid.

6. Textbook Committee, *Physiology of Sports National Textbook* (1983).

7. *Journal of the Wuhan Institute of Physical Education,* (No. 4, 1981).

Index

Table of Forms

BOOKS FROM YMAA

6 HEALING MOVEMENTS
101 REFLECTIONS ON TAI CHI CHUAN
A WOMAN'S QIGONG GUIDE
ADVANCING IN TAE KWON DO
ANCIENT CHINESE WEAPONS
ANALYSIS OF SHAOLIN CHIN NA 2ND ED.
ARTHRITIS RELIEF: CHINESE QIGONG FOR HEALING & PREVENTION, 3RD ED.
BACK PAIN RELIEF: CHINESE QIGONG FOR HEALING & PREVENTION 2ND ED
BAGUAZHANG
CARDIO KICKBOXING ELITE
CHIN NA IN GROUND FIGHTING
CHINESE FAST WRESTLING: THE ART OF SAN SHOU KUAI JIAO
CHINESE FITNESS: A MIND / BODY APPROACH
CHINESE TUI NA MASSAGE
COMPLETE CARDIOKICKBOXING
COMPREHENSIVE APPLICATIONS OF SHAOLIN CHIN NA
CONFLICT COMMUNICATION
DUKKHA: A SAM REEVES MARTIAL ARTS THRILLER
DUKKHA REVERB: A SAM REEVES MARTIAL ARTS THRILLER
DUKKHA UNLOADED: A SAM REEVES MARTIAL ARTS THRILLER
EIGHT SIMPLE QIGONG EXERCISES FOR HEALTH, 2ND ED.
ENZAN: THE FAR MOUNTAIN
ESSENCE OF SHAOLIN WHITE CRANE
ESSENCE OF TAIJI QIGONG, 2ND ED.
FACING VIOLENCE
FIGHTING ARTS
INSIDE TAI CHI
KATA AND THE TRANSMISSION OF KNOWLEDGE
LITTLE BLACK BOOK OF VIOLENCE
LIUHEBAFA FIVE CHARACTER SECRETS
MARTIAL ARTS ATHLETE
MARTIAL ARTS INSTRUCTION
MARTIAL WAY AND ITS VIRTUES
MEDITATIONS ON VIOLENCE
MIND/BODY FITNESS: A MIND / BODY APPROACH
THE MIND INSIDE TAI CHI
MUGAI RYU: THE CLASSICAL SAMURAI ART OF DRAWING THE SWORD
NATURAL HEALING WITH QIGONG: THERAPEUTIC QIGONG
NORTHERN SHAOLIN SWORD, 2ND ED.
OKINAWA'S COMPLETE KARATE SYSTEM: ISSHIN RYU

PRINCIPLES OF TRADITIONAL CHINESE MEDICINE
QIGONG FOR HEALTH & MARTIAL ARTS 2ND ED.
QIGONG FOR LIVING
QIGONG FOR TREATING COMMON AILMENTS
QIGONG MASSAGE —FUNDAMENTAL TECHNIQUES FOR HEALTH AND RELAXATION, 2ND ED.
QIGONG MEDITATION: EMBRYONIC BREATHING
QIGONG MEDITATION—SMALL CIRCULATION
QIGONG, THE SECRET OF YOUTH
QUIET TEACHER
ROOT OF CHINESE QIGONG, 2ND ED.
SHIN GI TAI—KARATE TRAINING FOR BODY, MIND, AND SPIRIT
SHIHAN TE: THE BUNKAI OF KATA
SIMPLIFIED TAI CHI CHUAN 24 & 48 POSTURES
SUNRISE TAI CHI
SURVIVING ARMED ASSAULTS
TAE KWON DO: THE KOREAN MARTIAL ART
TAEKWONDO BLACK BELT POOMSAE
TAEKWONDO: A PATH TO EXCELLENCE
TAEKWONDO: ANCIENT WISDOM FOR THE MODERN WARRIOR
TAEKWONDO: DEFENSES AGAINST WEAPONS
TAEKWONDO: SPIRIT AND PRACTICE
TAI CHI BALL QIGONG: FOR HEALTH AND MARTIAL ARTS
TAI CHI BOOK
TAI CHI CHIN NA: THE SEIZING ART OF TAI CHI CHUAN
TAI CHI CHUAN CLASSICAL YANG STYLE (REVISED EDITION)
TAI CHI CHUAN MARTIAL APPLICATIONS
TAI CHI CHUAN MARTIAL POWER
TAI CHI CONNECTIONS
TAI CHI DYNAMICS
TAI CHI QIGONG, 3RD ED.
TAI CHI SECRETS OF THE ANCIENT MASTERS
TAI CHI SECRETS OF THE WU & LI STYLES
TAI CHI SECRETS OF THE WU STYLE
TAI CHI SECRETS OF THE YANG STYLE
TAI CHI SWORD: CLASSICAL YANG STYLE
TAIJIQUAN THEORY OF DR. YANG, JWING-MING
TENGU: THE MOUNTAIN GOBLIN, A CONNOR BURKE MARTIAL ARTS THRILLER
TRADITIONAL CHINESE HEALTH SECRETS
TRADITIONAL TAEKWONDO
WESTERN HERBS FOR MARTIAL ARTISTS
XINGYIQUAN, 2ND ED.

DVDS FROM YMAA

ANALYSIS OF SHAOLIN CHIN NA
ADVANCED PRACTICAL CHIN NA IN DEPTH
BAGUAZHANG 1,2, & 3 —EMEI BAGUAZHANG
CHEN STYLE TAIJIQUAN
CHIN NA IN DEPTH COURSES 1: 4
CHIN NA IN DEPTH COURSES 5: 8
CHIN NA IN DEPTH COURSES 9: 12
EIGHT SIMPLE QIGONG EXERCISES FOR HEALTH
THE ESSENCE OF TAIJI QIGONG
FIVE ANIMAL SPORTS
INFIGHTING
KNIFE DEFENSE—TRADITIONAL TECHINIQUES AGAINST DAGGER
MERIDIAN QIGONG
NEIGONG FOR MARTIAL ARTS
QIGONG FOR HEALING
QIGONG MASSAGE—FUNDAMENTAL TECHNIQUES FOR HEALTH AND RELAXATION
SHAOLIN KUNG FU FUNDAMENTAL TRAINING 1&2
SHAOLIN LONG FIST KUNG FU: BASIC SEQUENCES
SHAOLIN SABER: BASIC SEQUENCES
SHAOLIN STAFF: BASIC SEQUENCES
SHAOLIN WHITE CRANE GONG FU BASIC TRAINING 1&2
SIMPLE QIGONG EXERCISES FOR ARTHRITIS RELIEF
SIMPLE QIGONG EXERCISES FOR BACK PAIN RELIEF
SIMPLIFIED TAI CHI CHUAN

SUNRISE TAI CHI
SUNSET TAI CHI
SWORD—FUNDAMENTAL TRAINING
TAI CHI ENERGY PATTERNS
TAIJI BALL QIGONG COURSES 1&2—16 CIRCLING AND 16 ROTATING PATTERNS
TAIJI BALL QIGONG COURSES 3&4—16 PATTERNS OF WRAP-COILING & APPLICATIONS
TAIJI MARTIAL APPLICATIONS: 37 POSTURES
TAIJI PUSHING HANDS 1&2—YANG STYLE SINGLE AND DOUBLE PUSHING HANDS
TAIJI PUSHING HANDS 3&4—MOVING SINGLE AND DOUBLE PUSH-ING HANDS
TAIJI SABER: THE COMPLETE FORM, QIGONG & APPLICATIONS
TAIJI & SHAOLIN STAFF - FUNDAMENTAL TRAINING
TAIJI YIN YANG STICKING HANDS
TAIJIQUAN CLASSICAL YANG STYLE
TAIJI SWORD, CLASSICAL YANG STYLE
UNDERSTANDING QIGONG 1: WHAT IS QI? • HUMAN QI CIRCULATORY SYSTEM
UNDERSTANDING QIGONG 2: KEY POINTS • QIGONG BREATHING
UNDERSTANDING QIGONG 3: EMBRYONIC BREATHING
UNDERSTANDING QIGONG 4: FOUR SEASONS QIGONG
UNDERSTANDING QIGONG 5: SMALL CIRCULATION
UNDERSTANDING QIGONG 6: MARTIAL QIGONG BREATHING
WHITE CRANE HARD & SOFT QIGONG
YANG TAI CHI FOR BEGINNERS

more products available from...
YMAA Publication Center, Inc. 楊氏東方文化出版中心
1-800-669-8892 • info@ymaa.com • www.ymaa.com

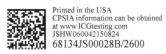

Printed in the USA
CPSIA information can be obtained
at www.ICGtesting.com
JSHW060042150824
68134JS00028B/2600